Springer
Tokyo
Berlin
Heidelberg
New York
Barcelona
Budapest
Hong Kong
London
Milan
Paris
Santa Clara
Singapore

T. Morimitsu

Cholesteatoma and Anterior Tympanotomy

With 82 Figures, Including 9 in Color

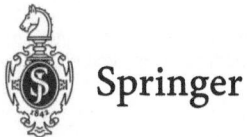 Springer

Tamotsu Morimitsu, M.D.
President
Miyazaki Medical College
5200 Kiyotake
Miyazaki, 889-16 Japan

ISBN-13: 978-4-431-68441-1   e-ISBN-13: 978-4-431-68439-8
DOI: 10.1007/978-4-431-68439-8

Cataloging-in-Publication Data applied for.

Printed on acid-free paper

Typesetting: Best-set Typesetter Ltd., Hong Kong

Preface

Acquired aural cholesteatoma poses a unique procedural dilemma with regard to pathogenetic research and theory building. Because cholesteatoma spontaneously occurs only in the poorly pneumatized human ear, its pathogenesis is specific to humans. Nonetheless, because of the ethical questions surrounding human experimentation, pathogenetic study has almost exclusively involved nonhuman subjects. Indeed, attempts have failed in almost all animal experiments except with the gerbil, and even here experimental designs have been improbable compared with human cholesteatoma. Cholesteatoma in the gerbil is useful, therefore, only for the study of pathology and not for human pathogenesis.

I hold that the pathogenesis of cholesteatoma will be understood by studying the cholesteatomatous ear, that is, the malpneumatized ear of the human. The anatomical difference between the normal and malpneumatized ear is a probable cause of cholesteatoma. This difference may be found clinically in facial nerve decompression and cholesteatoma surgery, as, for example, facial nerve palsy occurs usually in the normal, well-pneumatized ear. Of course, conventional animal experimentation will not confirm this clinical difference since there is no ideal animal model for the poorly pneumatized human ear.

Present surgical techniques for cholesteatoma vary greatly according to individual otosurgeon's opinion. The most extreme difference of opinion is focused on whether to remove the external ear canal wall. Normally, the best option would be not to remove the canal wall if cholesteatoma recurrence can be prevented. Simply put, recurrence of cholesteatoma comes about when its cause has not been removed during primary surgery.

In my own practice, I have operated on recurrent cases, hypothesizing that there is a higher likelihood of finding the pathogenesis by way of secondary surgery. With this view I have developed a new surgical technique, namely, anterior tympanotomy. With anterior tympanotomy, recurrence rates have decreased significantly. Furthermore, I have concluded that the osseous tympanic diaphragm created by malpneumatization at the supratubal recess after birth is the actual pathogenesis of cholesteatoma. This conclusion has been strengthened by anatomical and embryological studies conducted by members of the ENT

Department at Miyazaki Medical College, as well as by histological research at the Minnesota Temporal Bone Bank.

My theory on the pathogenesis of cholesteatoma is derived from 40 years of surgical experience and 8 years of clinical results on anterior tympanotomy. These results were reported at the 92nd Annual Congress of the Oto-rhino-laryngological Society of Japan (1991). This volume presents that research in English, with additional reports of results of anterior tympanotomy obtained since 1991.

My purpose here is to demonstrate reasons for you to consider anterior tympanotomy combined with the canal-up method in cases of cholesteatoma. In this way, you may help complete this work on acquired aural cholesteatoma and help confirm its benefits clinically.

I would like to express sincere thanks to the colleagues listed below, as well as to G. Hansen in Minneapolis in preparing this manuscript.

In the anatomical study of temporal bones: Kouji Makino, M.D., Kouji Matsuura, M.D., and Yoshihiro Ueki, M.D.

In the embryological study of temporal bones: Yuichiro Adachi, M.D., and Akihiko Naichu, Ph.D.

In the histopathological study of temporal bones: Tetsuya Tono, M.D., and Satoshi Miyanaga, M.D.

In the electron microscopical study of temporal bones: Tomoyuki Nagai, M.D., and Kiyo Kano, M.D.

Audiological studies: Yasuaki Ushisako, Ph.D., and Eiji Kato, Ph.D.

Radiological studies: Hirokazu Kawano, M.D., Kiyo Kano, M.D., and Tetsuya Tono, M.D.

Clinical studies: Ichiro Natsumoto, M.D., Yoichiro Ochiai, M.D., Tomoyuki Nagai, M.D., Midori Nagai, M.D., Shizuo Komune, M.D., Shuichi Okada, M.D., Masami Takahashi, M.D., Kunitoshi Enatsu, M.D., Yoshimi Mitani, M.D., Minoru Ide, M.D., Kouji Makino, M.D., Tetsuya Tono, M.D., Setsuko Hidaka, M.D., Yuichiro Adachi, M.D., Fujihiko Kasano, M.D., Mikiko Fukiyama, M.D., Kazuki Saku, M.D., Akitoshi Hayashi, M.D., Kiyo Kano, M.D., Meiko Asami, M.D., Satoshi Miyanaga, M.D., Hirokazu Kawano, M.D., Atsushi Haruta, M.D., Miharu Imuta, M.D., Yoshihiro Ueki, M.D., Kouji Matsuura, M.D., Yuko Nagata, M.D., Yukiyo Hara, M.D., Katsuhiro Toyama, M.D., Keiji Matsuda, M.D., Kouji Tsuboi, M.D., Kouji Torihara, M.D., Masayuki Sadanaga, M.D., Masami Shimozono, M.D., Junko Inaba, M.D., Jiro Ichihara, M.D., Hiroto Osako, M.D., Kenichi Horinouchi, M.D., Yoko Tsuboi, M.D., Yasuko Ninomiya, M.D., Mika Takenaka, M.D., Hiroshi Makimoto, M.D., Miki Morimoto, M.D., Ken Ito, M.D., Takashi Nabekura, M.D., and Misako Nishiura, M.D.

During the preparation of this book I was a professor in the department of Otorhinolaryngology, of which it was my privilege to serve as Chairman, at Miyazaki Medical College. The support of members of the faculty of my academic department is greatly appreciated, as is support from the following other departments of Miyazaki Medical College: Radiology, Oral Surgery, Second Anatomy, and First and Second Pathology.

I would also like to acknowledge the individual support of Naomasa Okamoto, M.D., former President of Miyazaki Medical College, and Yoshiteru Goto, M.D., of our college's Electron Microscope Center; Yukio Sato, M.D., and Toshimasu Ri, M.D., of the Hiroshima Atomic Bomb Institute; M.M. Paparella, M.D., Tetsuo Morizono, M.D., and Noriko Morizono, Ph.D., of the Faculty of Medicine at the University of Minnesota; Kenji Aimi, M.D., of the Faculty of Medicine at the University of Illinois; and C. Jansen, M.D., of Gummerbach, Germany.

Finally, I thank my wife Yasuko and our children, Yukiko and Takashi.

January 1997

Tamotsu Morimitsu, M.D.
President
Miyazaki Medical College

Contents

Chapter 6. Computed Tomography of the Cholesteatomatous Ear

Chapter 7. Pathogenesis of Cholesteatoma

Chapter 1
Introduction

In this book, two types of primary acquired cholesteatoma are discussed: one is attic cholesteatoma, which develops when Shrapnell's membrane (the pars flaccida) retracts into Prussak's space and then into the epitympanic cavity, and the other is adhesive cholesteatoma, which develops from retraction pockets into the epitympanic cavity when the tympanic membrane adheres to the promontory. Bezold (1889) stated that attic cholesteatoma is the result of occlusion of the eustachian tube that causes retraction pockets of Shrapnell's membrane in which the keratinizing layer of epithelium desquamates. His retraction pocket theory has received widespread acceptance (Tos et al. 1988).

There are, however, some clinical facts inconsistent with Bezold's theory of tubal occlusion. For instance, Honjo (1988) reported that the eustachian tube, in 77% of cases of retraction cholesteatoma, had normal or reduced opening pressure. Furthermore, there are many cases of attic retraction with perforation of the pars tensa in which negative pressure in the tympanic cavity cannot occur. Therefore, we must assume the existence of a partition between the mesotympanum and epitympanum that may cause negative pressure locally in the epitympanum followed by retraction of Shrapnell's membrane without tubal occlusion.

Wittmaack (1933) found that hyperplastic embryonic mucoperiosteum in the attic could cause attic bloc and then retraction pockets and that this hyperplastic mucosa causes poorly pneumatized temporal bone, in which attic cholesteatoma is usually seen. Proctor (1964) emphasized the relatively small communications (the anterior and posterior tympanic isthmuses) between mesotympanum and epitympanum, which are prone to occlusion by edematous mucosa, thus closing off aeration of the mastoid cells and causing negative pressure in the epitympanum.

Since 1965, I have operated on small cholesteatomas using the intact canal wall method, later combined with posterior tympanotomy (Jansen 1967; Sheehy and Patterson 1967). I have been forced to reoperate in about 25% of these cases because of recurrent cholesteatoma. The following observations from surgical findings in these reoperations reflect my surgical methodology: (1) eradication of cholesteatoma matrix alone is ineffective against recurrence of cholesteatoma;

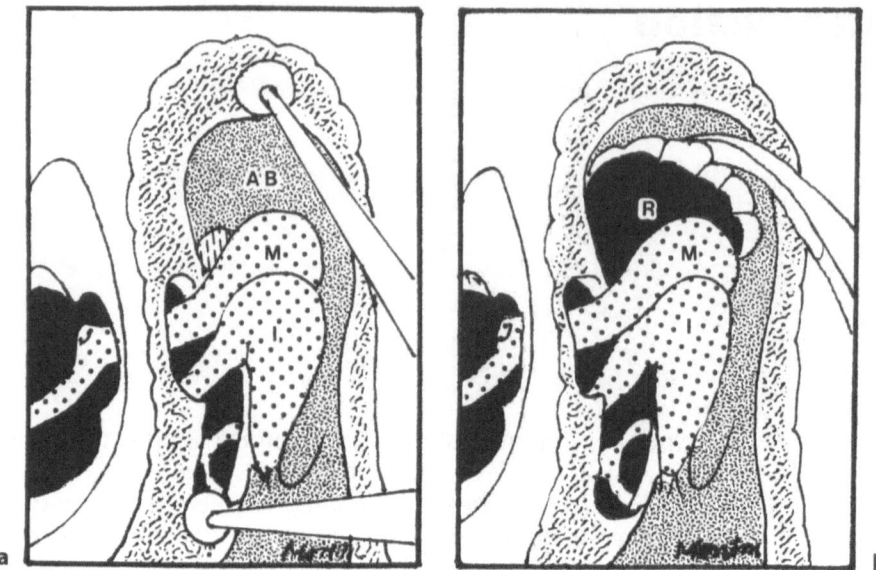

Fig. 1–1a,b. Anterior tympanotomy. **a** Status directly before anterior tympanotomy and after posterior tympanotomy. *AB*, anterior attic bony plate; *M*, malleus; *I*, incus. **b** Anterior tympanotomy in progress with a curved chisel. *R*, supratubal recess

(2) postoperative patency of a formerly closed tympanic isthmus is very difficult to maintain; (3) there is a high incidence of reclosure of ventilating routes made by posterior tympanotomy; and (4) a new ventilating route must be made to the epitympanum from the eustachian tube other than the tympanic isthmus or the route made by posterior tympanotomy.

In 1983, I found (serendipitously) a large cavity after removal of a bony plate in front of the malleal head. There I could obtain a wide ventilating route to the eustachian tube in case of reoperation. I then tried this technique in all primary and reoperated cases and got excellent postoperative results. This bony plate had already been reported by Hoshino and Suzuki (1978), who called it the anterior attic bony plate. In 1985, I reported on this surgical technique, calling it anterior tympanotomy because the anterior tympanic cavity is opened in this procedure (Fig. 1–1).

Our clinical results (Morimitsu et al. 1983, 1984, 1989a, 1989b and Morimitsu 1991) using anterior tympanotomy in surgery for cholesteatoma, which have been accumulated for more than 10 years, show that the rate of recurrence of cholesteatoma has decreased significantly with use of this technique. In my experience, it seems correct to judge the clinical processes in recurrent cholesteatoma to be the same as those in primary cholesteatoma. Furthermore, it appears that the pathogenesis of cholesteatoma must be related to the sites removed by anterior tympanotomy, i.e., the supratubal recess and the anterior attic bony plate, important parts of the tympanic diaphragm.

In this volume, the pathogenesis of acquired attic and adhesive cholesteatomas are explained by reference to results obtained in basic anatomical studies of the temporal bone and in surgery for cholesteatoma combined with anterior tympanotomy.

References

Bezold F (1889) Cholesteatoma, Perforation der Membrane flaccida und Tubenkatarrh. Z Ohrenheilk 20:5–21

Honjo I (1988) Evstachian tube and middle ear diseases. Springer-Verlag, Berlin Heidelberg New York Tokyo

Hoshino T, Suzuki J (1978) Anterior attic wall anatomy. Arch Otolaryngol 104:588–590

Jansen C (1967) Posteriore Tympanotomie: Zugang zum Mittelohr mit Erhaltung des ausseren Gehoehrgangs. Arch Otorhinolaryngol 188:2–6

Morimitsu T (1991) Etiology of middle ear cholesteatoma (in Japanese with English abstract). Otolog Fukuoka 37:271–405

Morimitsu T, Matsumoto I, Nagai T, Komune S, Enatsu K, Ide M (1983) Anterior tympanotomy against recurrence of cholesteatoma. In: Proceedings, 5th Asia-Oceania Congress, Seoul, October 9–14

Morimitsu T, Matsumoto I, Nagai T, Komune S, Enatsu K, Ide M (1984) Anterior tympanotomy. Clin Otol Jpn 11:270–271

Morimitsu T, Matsumoto I, Nagai T, Ide M, Makino K, Tono T (1989a) Long-term results of anterior tympanotomy for cholesteatoma. In: Tos M, Thomsen J, Peitersen E (eds) Cholesteatoma and mastoid surgery. Kugler & Ghedini, Amsterdam, pp 875–880

Morimitsu T, Matsumoto I, Nagai T, Nagai M, Ide M, Makino K, Tono T, Adachi Y, Kasano F, Fukiyama M, Hayashi A (1989b) Pathogenesis of cholesteatoma based on clinical results of anterior tympanotomy. Auris Nasus Larynx (Tokyo) 16(suppl 1):9–14

Proctor B (1964) The development of the middle ear spaces and their surgical significance. J Laryngol 78:631–648

Sheehy JL, Patterson ME (1967) Intact canal wall tympanoplasty with mastoidectomy. Laryngoscope 70:1502–1542

Tos M, Stangerup S-E, Larsen PL, Siim C, Hvid G, Andreassen UK (1988) The relationship between secretory otitis and cholesteatoma. In: Tos M, Thomsen J, Peitersen E (eds) Cholesteatoma and mastoid surgery. Kugler & Ghedini, Amsterdam, pp 325–330

Wittmaack K (1933) Wie entsteht ein genuines Cholesteatoma? Arch Ohren Nasen Kehlkopf 137:306

Chapter 2
Anatomical Studies

2.1 Normal Adult Temporal Bone

2.1.1 The Protympanum of the Tympanic Cavity

The tympanic cavity may be divided into five parts: protympanum, meso-tympanum, retrotympanum, hypotympanum, and epitympanum. The anterior margin of the protympanum is the aperture of the eustachian tube, and its posterior margin is the line projected from it onto the promontory of the anterior margin of the tympanic anulus. The protympanum includes a part of the osseous eustachian tube, the semicanal of the tensor tympani muscle, the supratubal recess, and the cochleariform process with the tensor tympani tendon. It covers the internal carotid artery, the cochlea, the geniculate ganglion, and the petrous portion of the facial nerve (Fig. 2–1). Although it is difficult to draw definite borderlines separating each of the parts of the tympanum, there is a clear border-line between the pro-/mesotympanum and the epitympanum, called the tympanic diaphragm.

2.1.2 The Tympanic Diaphragm and the Tympanic Isthmus

The name tympanic diaphragm was introduced by French anatomists Chatellier and Lemoine in 1946. The "diaphragme interattico-tympanique" in a newborn baby reported by them is shown in Fig. 2–2. It lies nearly horizontally from the tensor tympani mucosal fold to the stapedial tendon. They pointed out an open-ing 2.5 mm in diameter in the tympanic diaphragm, which Wullstein (1984) called the second bottleneck in the middle-ear space (the eustachian tube is the first bottleneck).

Proctor (1989) reported that the attic floor (tympanic diaphragm) is made up of the malleal head and neck, the body and short crus of the incus, the anterior malleal ligament, the lateral and medial incudal folds, the fold of the tensor, and even the plica stapedius and the membrane obturatoria. There are two small openings in the tympanic diaphragm: the anterior tympanic isthmus, between the tensor tympani tendon and the stapes, and the posterior tympanic isthmus, be-

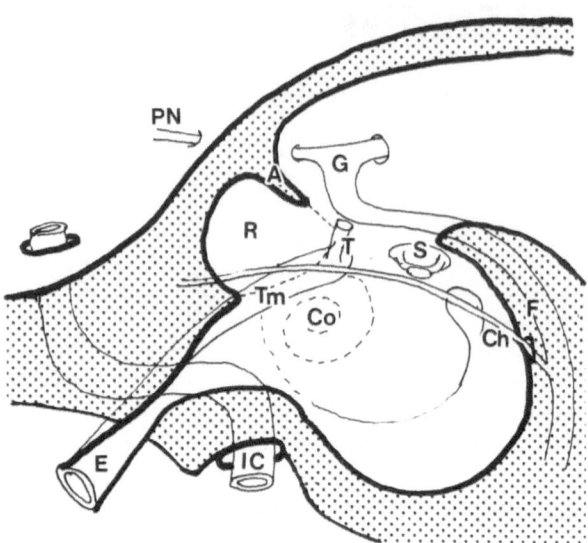

Fig. 2–1. The protympanum and its parts. *A*, anterior attic bony plate; *Tm*, semicanal of tensor tympani muscle; *R*, supratubal recess; *T*, tensor tympani tendon and cochleariformis process; *IC*, internal carotid artery; *E*, eustachian tube; *Co*, cochlea; *G*, geniculate ganglion; *F*, facial nerve; *Ch*, chorda tympani; *PN*, superior petrosal nerve; *S*, stapes

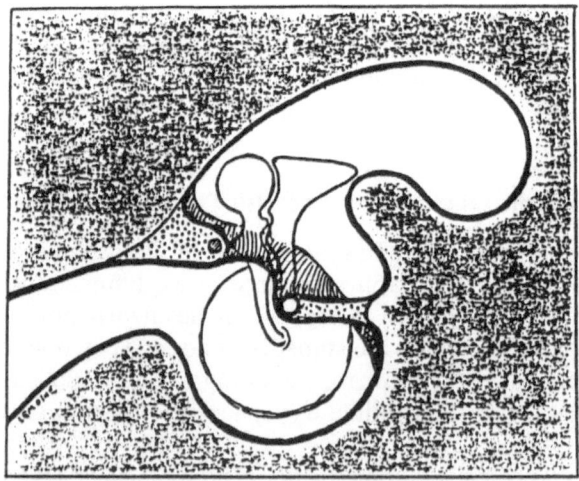

Fig. 2–2. Diaphragme interattico-tympanique, reported by Chatellier and Lemoine (1946). (With permission)

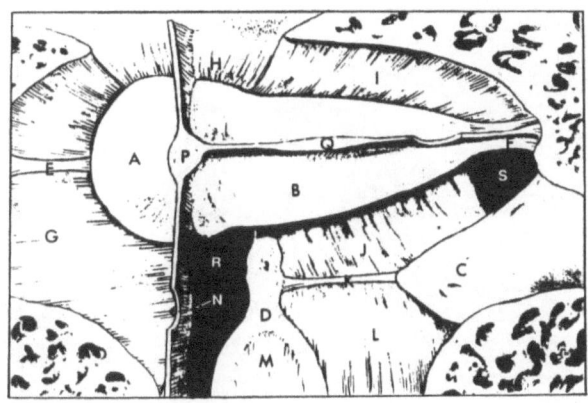

Fig. 2–3. Floor of the attic, reported by Proctor (1989). *R*, anterior tympanic isthmus; *S*, posterior tympanic isthmus; *A*, malleus head; *B*, body of incus; *C*, pyramidal eminence; *D*, stapes; *E*, anterior mallear ligament; *F*, posterior incudal ligament; *G*, tensor fold; *H*, lateral mallear fold; *I*, lateral incudal fold; *J*, medial incudal fold; *K*, stapedal tendon; *L*, plica stapedis; *M*, membrana obturatoria stapedis; *N*, incisura tensoris; *O*, superior mallear fold; *P*, superior mallear ligament. (With permission)

tween the medial incudal fold and the bony posterior tympanic wall (Fig. 2–3). Proctor described further that inflammatory swelling of the mucosa and mucosal folds can easily close the tympanic isthmuses, blocking the flow of air and exudate between the attic above and the mesotympanum below. His theory is, however, true only in poorly pneumatized ears and in newborns. In well-pneumatized ears, there is a ventilation route through the supratubal recess (STR route) as well as through the tympanic isthmus (isthmic route).

2.1.3 The Supratubal Recess

The supratubal recess (STR) is an area of the protympanum that protrudes upward from the eustachian tube over the tensor tympani semicanal and is located in front of the attic, forming the most anterior part of the tympanic diaphragm. Names for this recess include many synonyms: supratubal space (Proctor 1989), sinus epitympani (Wigand and Trillsch 1974), anterior epitympanic cell (Gacek 1980), anterior epitympanic space (Hoshino 1988), anterior epitympanic recess (Schuknecht and Gulya 1986; Sheehy 1979), supratubal recess (Horn et al. 1986). We use the term supratubal recess; it seems most reasonable. At its superior boundary with the epitympanum, there is a bony plate called by Hoshino and Suzuki (1978) the anterior attic bony plate (Fig. 2–4), by W. House (cited from Horn et al. 1986) the cog, and by Wullstein (1984) the crista anterior. Its inferior boundary with the eustachian tube is the semicanal of the tensor tympani.

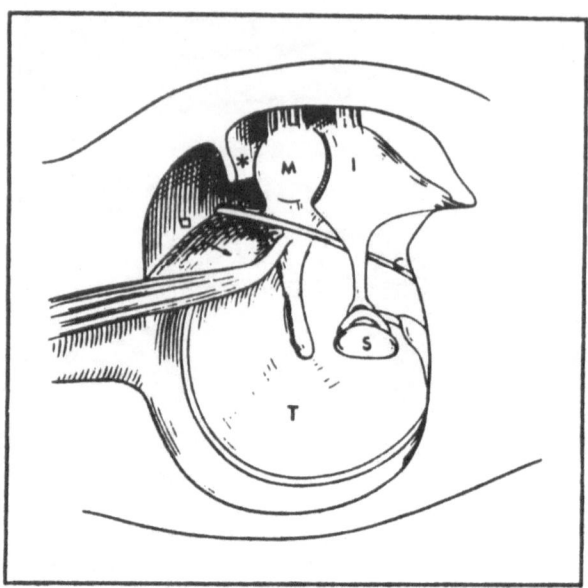

Fɪɢ. 2–4. Anterior attic bony plate, reported by Hoshino and Suzuki (1978). Anterior attic bony plate (*asterisk*) separates attic from supratubal space (*square*), which is delimited from eustachian tube orifice by tensor tympani fold (*arrow*). *M*, malleus; *I*, incus; *S*, stapes; *T*, tympanum. (With permission)

2.1.4 Anatomical Studies of the Supratubal Recess

In our laboratory, 34 normal adult temporal bones were studied; 26 were cut sagittally parallel to the tympanic membrane using a diamond bandsaw (Exakt, Hamburg, Germany), 6 were cut axially at the tegmen tympani, and 2 were cut coronally, crossing the eustachian tube. Each cut surface was observed under a surgical microscope, photographed, and then measured at determined points using a slide caliper. The temporal bones were classified into three groups according to the grade of pneumatization shown: pneumatized (14 ears), well pneumatized (15 ears), and extremely well pneumatized (5 ears).

Figure 2–5 shows photographs of sagittally sectioned bones cut at the level of the eardrum. In Fig. 2–5a, the anterior attic mucosal fold (Am) is transparently thin and perforated and partly adhered at the malleal head. The anterior attic bony plate (Ab) is short, and the tensor tympani mucosal fold (Tm) is almost totally perforated. This type of supratubal recess is classified as the "medial type."

In Fig. 2–5b, the anterior attic mucosal fold shows a round perforation, and the anterior attic bony plate is rudimentary. The tensor tympani mucosal fold is semitransparent with a thick margin and is not perforated. The bony plate near the tensor tympani is just like a ledge. The partitions are close together and located more superiorly, so that the supratubal recess is narrow. This type of supratubal recess is called the superior type.

In Fig. 2–5c, a part of the anterior attic bony plate touches on the malleal head. The tensor tympani mucosal fold is semitransparent and perforated. The tegmen tympani shows a "double layer" (Dt), so called because of extreme pneumatization. The STR is large. In Fig. 2–5d, the anterior attic bony plate is like a frame, and its mucosal fold is absent. The mucosal fold of the tensor tympani is small and perforated. An extra bony plate (Ex) similar to the anterior attic bony plate is visible over the original plate.

Figure 2–6 shows views of axial cuts from the tegmen tympani. In Fig. 2–6a, the anterior attic bony plate, the large supratubal recess (R), the posterior tympanic isthmus (Ti), and Prussak's space (P) are visible. The tensor tympani mucosal fold is almost totally perforated. Figure 2–6b is the same specimen as in Fig. 2–6a, but viewed a little more anteriorly. The thin, but not perforated, anterior attic mucosal fold is clearly visible. It attaches at the tensor tympani tendon (T). In Fig. 2–6c, the anterior attic bony plate and its mucosal fold (attached partly to the malleal head) are visible. The tensor tympani mucosal fold is thick and not perforated.

Figure 2–7 shows coronal sections. In Fig. 2–7a, the anterior attic bony plate looks like a cog, and the anterior attic mucosal fold is mostly absent or is rudimentary around the tensor tympani tendon. In Fig. 2–7b, the anterior attic bony plate and its mucosal fold are equally rudimentary. The superior and lateral malleal folds (Ms and Ml), Prussak's space (P), Schrapnell's membrane (Sh), Troeltsch's space (Tr), and the tensor tympani tendon are clearly visible.

2.1.5 Measurements of the Supratubal Recess and Related Structures

The results from our study of measurements of the STR and related structures in 32 temporal bones are as follows. The anterior attic bony plate existed in 30 of 32 ears (94%). It was located superiorly in 32%, inferiorly in 13%, and centrally in 55%. As shown in Fig. 2–8, its length (D) ranged from 0.6 to 1.7 mm, with an average of 1.2 mm. Its thickness at the base (C) ranged from 0.3 to 1.6 mm, with an average of 1.1 mm. Its width ranged from 0.9 to 2.9 mm, with an average of 1.5 mm. The distance to the malleal head (A) ranged from 0.8 to 2.2 mm, with an average of 1.4 mm. There was no correlation between the size of the bony plate and the grade of pneumatization.

The anterior attic mucosal fold existed in 18 of 34 ears (52%), and its mean length and width were 1.9 and 1.7 mm, respectively. The ratio between the area of the bony plate and the area of the mucosal fold was 1.0:1.8. Because of possible bone loss in cutting the specimens, these sizes may actually be a little larger in vivo. The angle between this mucosal fold and the tensor tympani mucosal fold averaged 34°. In eight ears, an extra mucosal fold was observed under the anterior attic mucosal fold, stretching from the tegmen to the tensor tympani tendon.

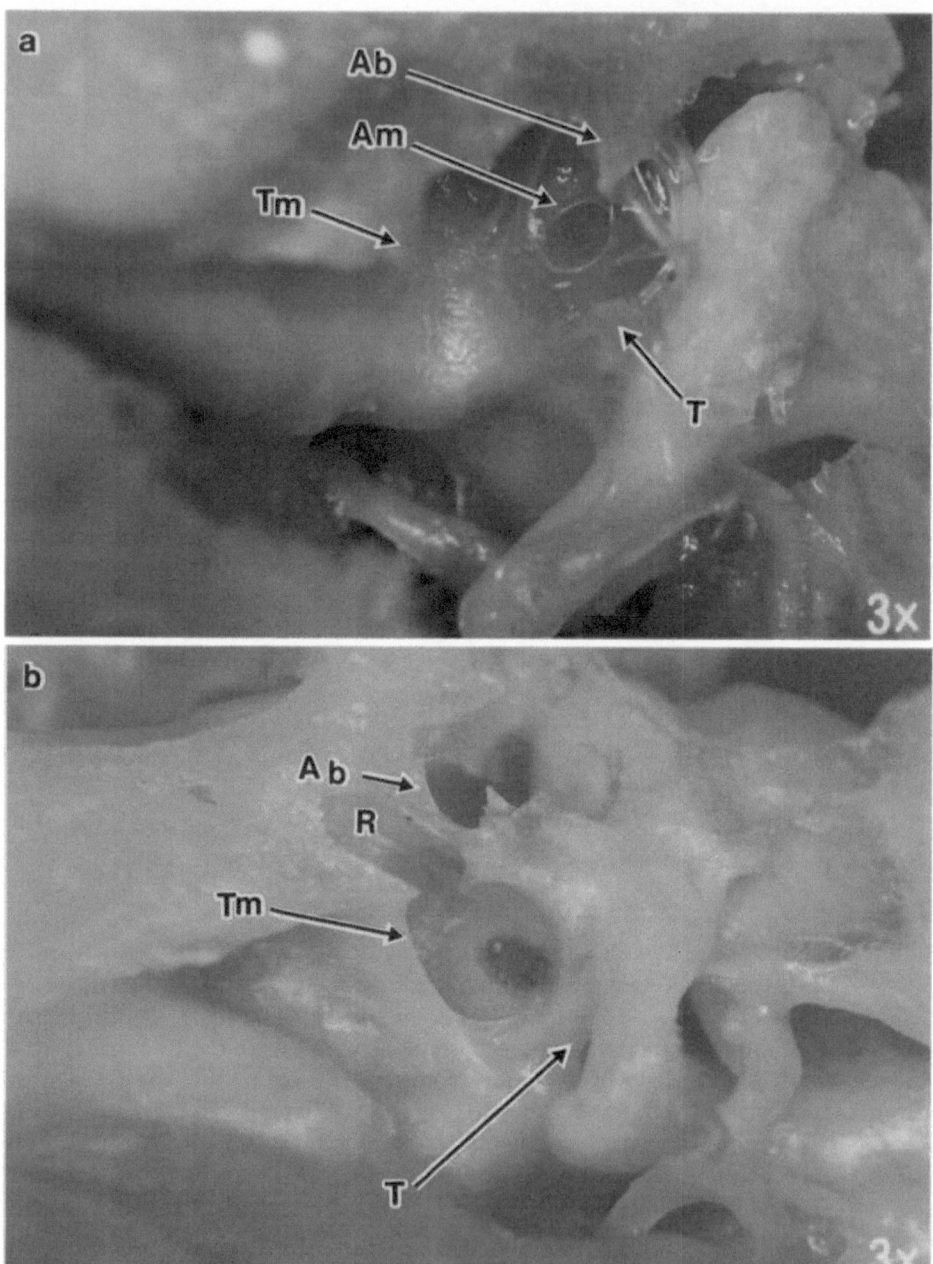

FIG. 2–5a–d. Sagittal sections at the line of the eardrum (see text). *Ab*, anterior attic bony plate; *Am*, anterior attic mucosal fold; *Tm*, tensor tympani mucosal fold; *T*, tensor tympani tendon; *R*, supratubal recess; *Dt*, so-called double-laid tegmen tympani; *Ex*, extra bony plate. ×3, ×2

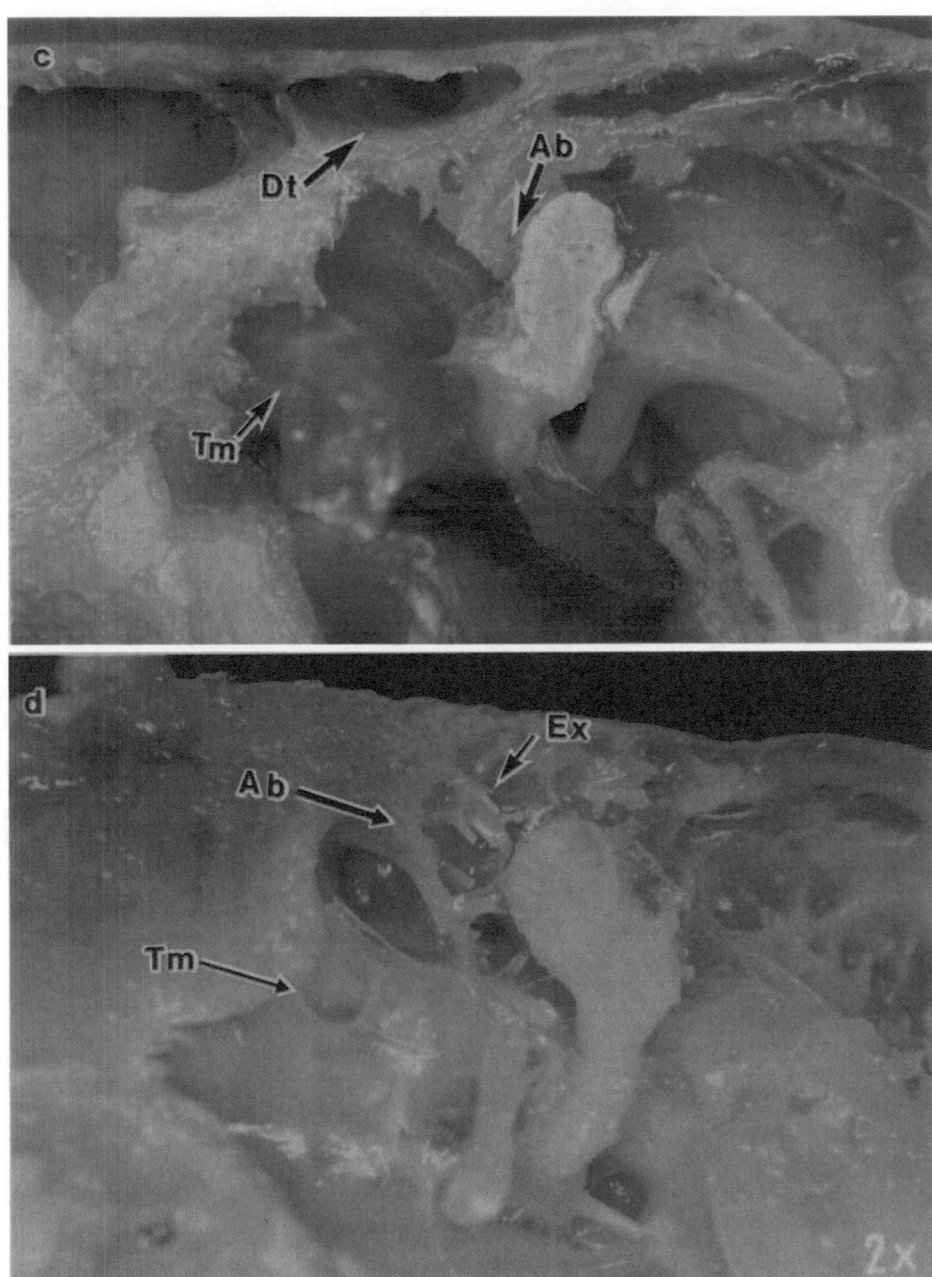

FIG. 2-5a-d. *Continued*

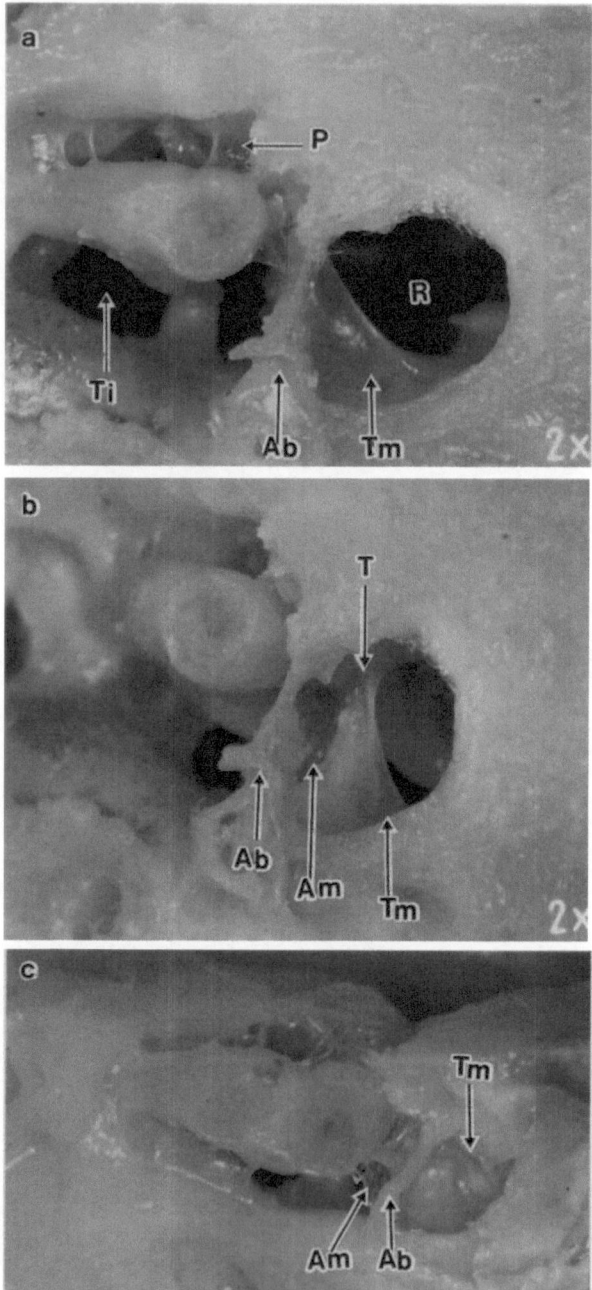

Fig. 2–6a–c. Axial sections at the level of the tegmen tympani (see text). *Ab*, anterior attic bony plate; *Am*, anterior attic mucosal fold; *Tm*, tensor tympani mucosal fold; *T*, tensor tympani tendon; *Ti*, posterior tympanic isthmus; *P*, Prussak's space; *R*, supratubal recess

FIG. 2–7a,b. Coronal sections at the level of the supratubal recess (**a**) and the tensor tympani tendon (**b**). *Ab*, anterior attic bony plate; *Am*, anterior attic mucosal fold; *Ms*, superior mallear ligament; *Ml*, lateral mallear ligament; *T*, tensor tympani tendon; *P*, Prussak's space; *Tr*, Troeltsch's space; *Sh*, Shrapnell's membrane

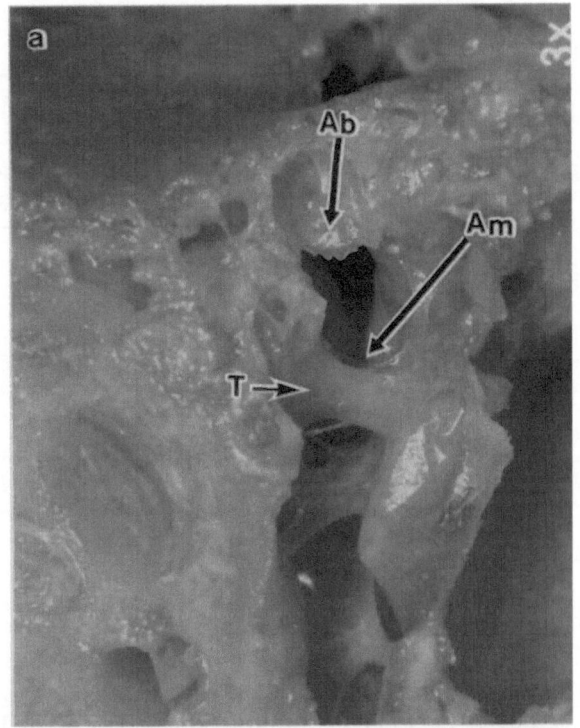

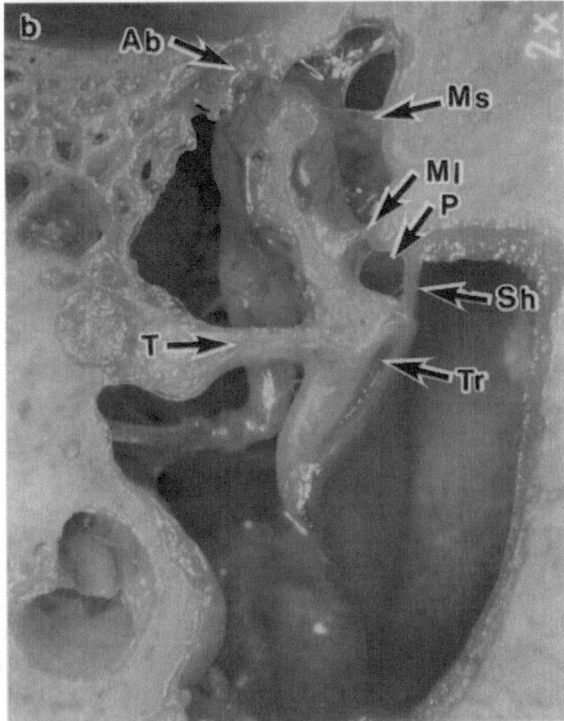

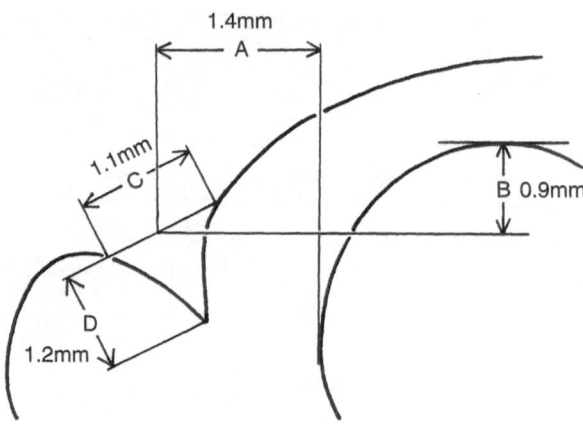

Fig. 2–8. Measurements of anterior attic bony plates and their average values. *A*, distance from the center of the bony plate to the mallear head; *B*, level of the mallear head from the center of the bony plate; *C*, thickness of the base of the bony plate; *D*, length of the anterior attic bony plate

The mucosal fold and bony plate of the tensor tympani, existed in 31 of 34 ears (91%), even though it was rudimentary in some ears. This fold was thicker than the other folds; its mean length and width were 2.4 and 2.0 mm, respectively. In 22 of the 31 ears (71%), the fold was perforated. The perforation was large in 17, medium sized in 3, and small (less than one-third of the mucosal fold) in 2 ears. There was no correlation between the size of the perforation and the degree of pneumatization (of the middle-ear space). In 2 of the 9 nonperforated folds, a thinner area was observed that appeared similar to a regenerated area of perforated eardrum. In 4 ears, the attached part of this fold at the anterior bony wall projected clearly, like a ledge; we called this ledge the tensor tympani bony plate. The angle between the mucosal fold of the tensor tympani and its bony plate, on the one hand, or the semicanal of the tensor tympani on the other, ranged from 0° to 50°, with an average of 27.5°. There was no correlation between this angle and the degree of pneumatization.

The supratubal recess is divided into two parts, the superior and the inferior recess, by the tensor tympani mucosal fold (Fig. 2–9). In our study, the size of the superior recess (A and A′) averaged 1.8 × 2.7 mm. These recesses were large in 15 ears, medium-sized in 8, and small in 8 ears. Sizes of the inferior recess (B and B′) averaged 2.0 × 2.7 mm. They were large in 9 ears, medium-sized in 9, and small in 11. Three ears had no inferior recess; the tensor tympani mucosal fold was parallel to the semicanal of the tensor tympani. The size of the superior recess and the degree of pneumatization are in proportion to each other; i.e., the larger the recess, the better the pneumatization. On the other hand, the size of the inferior recess does not correlate with the degree of pneumatization. In 4 of 28 temporal bones in our study, peritubal cells were observed, but they had no direct communication to the recess.

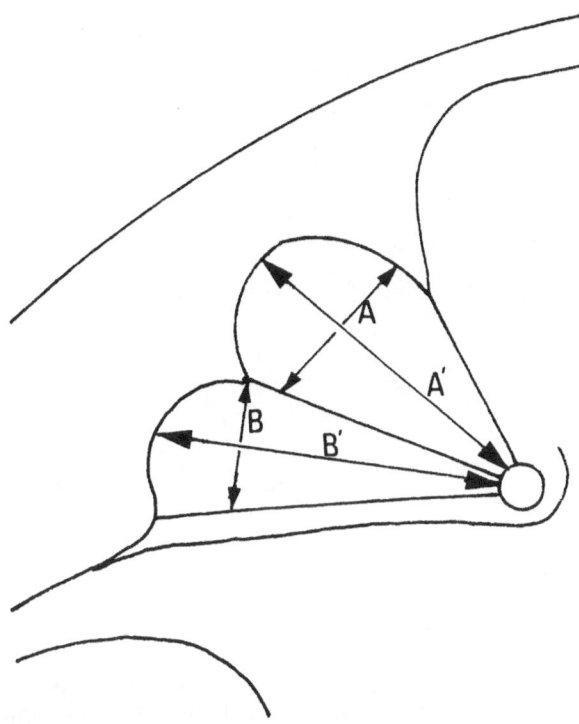

FIG. 2–9. Measurements of the supratubal recess. A and A', length and width of the superior supratubal recess; B and B', length and width of the inferior supratubal recess

Regarding other measurements in the epitympanum, the distance between the malleal head and the tegmen tympani could be measured exactly in 16 ears. The longest was 1.7 mm and the shortest 0.0 mm, averaging 0.7 mm, with no correlation with pneumatization. The thickness of the tegmen tympani was measured in 19 ears; the thickest was 4.0 mm and the thinnest 1.9 mm, with an average of 1.7 mm. Thicknesses for the group were 1.4, 1.9, and 2.1 mm, respectively, in parallel with the grades of pneumatization. A double layer was observed in the tegmen in 3 ears with extremely good pneumatization.

Figure 2–10 shows our final view of the tympanic diaphragm and its ventilation routes in well-pneumatized ears. The upper border of the STR consists of the anterior attic bony plate and its mucosal fold, and the lower border consists of the bony plate and mucosal fold of the tensor tympani. Both folds are very often perforated. In our study, the anterior attic bony plate and mucosal fold existed in 94% and 52% of all cases, respectively. The mucosal fold was perforated in 47%. On the other hand, the bony plate and mucosal fold of the tensor tympani existed in 1% and 91%, respectively. The tensor tympani mucosal fold was perforated in 70% of all cases. Both mucosal folds occurred in only 20% of all cases. In 94% of the specimens studied, one or the other of these mucosal folds was perforated, so

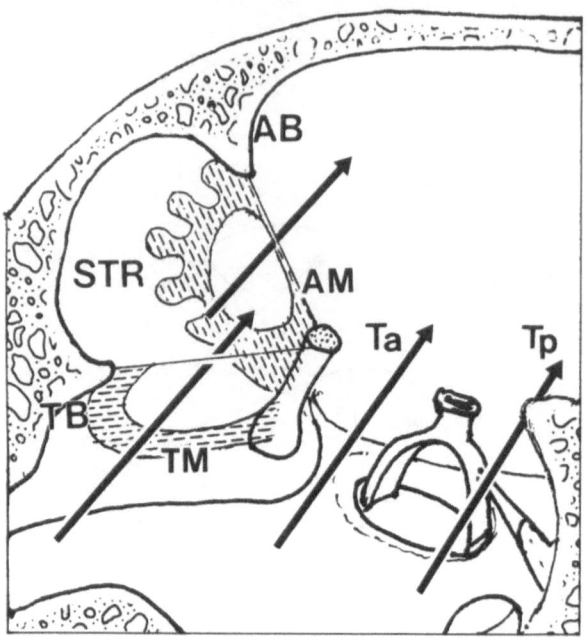

Fɪɢ. 2–10. Tympanic diaphragm and its ventilation routes in well-pneumatized ear. *AB*, anterior attic bony plate; *AM*, anterior attic mucosal fold; *TB*, tensor tympani bony plate; *TM*, tensor tympani mucosal fold; *Ta*, anterior tympanic isthmus; *Tp*, posterior tympanic isthmus; *STR*, supratubal recess

we concluded that ventilation from the eustachian tube into the epitympanum is possible through the STR in ways other than through the tympanic isthmuses in normally pneumatized adult ears.

2.2 Embryonal Temporal Bone

There are some reports on development of the tympanic cavity in humans (Proctor 1964; Ars 1986; Declau 1989; Shimizu 1987). No precise reports could be found, however, concerning development of the supratubal recess. We performed embryological studies of the middle ear cleft using a three-dimensional graphic reconstruction. For materials, we used bilateral fetal ears at 3 and 6 months of intrauterine development, and one ear each at 4, 5, 8, 9, and 10 months of intrauterine development, for a total of nine ears. All were from fetuses without definite abnormalities in the face or limbs. The duration of gestation was determined from the size of the head.

Our temporal bones were refixed in 10% formalin, decalcified with trichloracetic acid (TCA), then embedded in celloidin. The embedded specimens were marked for three-dimensional reconstruction, then sliced in 40 µm thicknesses using a microtome (TU-213, Yamato, Saitama, Japan), and stained with hematoxylin and eosin. We traced the following structures from projections of serial sections on an enlarging projector (UP-350, Olympas, Tokyo): the tympanic cavity, the eustachian tube, the ossicles, mesenchymal tissue, the facial

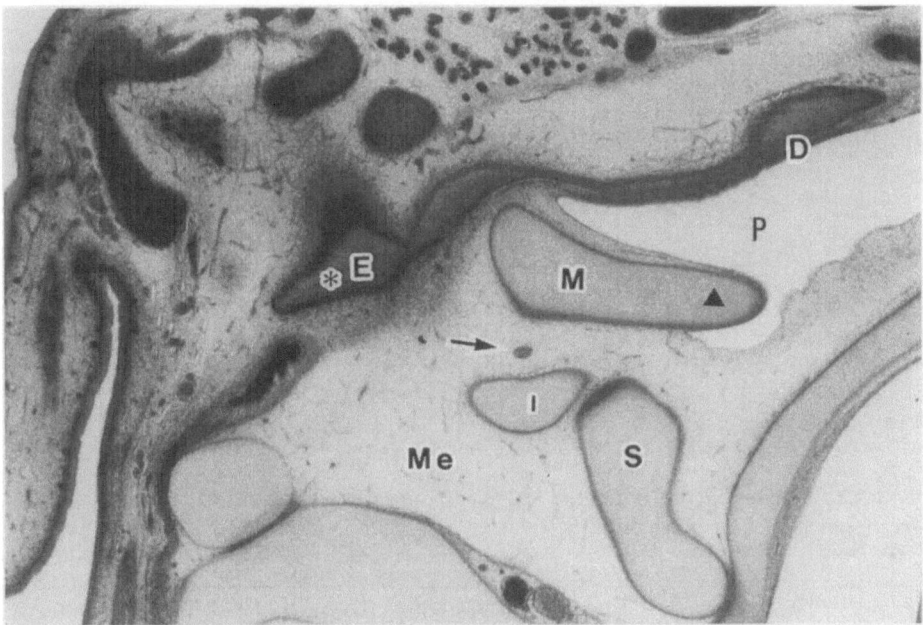

Fig. 2–11. Tympanic space at 3 months gestation. *P*, pouch from the epipharynx; *M*, malleus; *E*, meatal plate; *D*, eardrum; *I*, incus; *S*, stapes; *Me*, mesenchymal tissue around the ossicles; *triangle*, malleus handle; *asterisk*, meatal plate. *Arrow* indicates the chorda tympani

nerve, the tensor tympani muscle, the external ear canal, and the mucosal folds. The tracings were input into a computer (TRI-file, Ratocc, Tokyo, and Spicca, Abionics, Tokyo, Japan) using a television camera. The data were reconstructed three dimensionally and displayed on an oscilloscope with D-SCAN GR4416 (Seiko, Tokyo).

Some significant specimens are discussed here. Figure 2–11 shows the tympanic cavity at 3 months gestation. A simple pouch reaches from the epipharynx around the malleus body in the mesenchymal tissue. The external meatus is still the meatal plate, without a lumen (E). The eardrum (D), however, can already be recognized beside the pouch. The arrow indicates a nerve, probably the chorda tympani. At 5 months gestation (Fig. 2–12), ossification of the malleus and the incus is still in progress, and cartilaginous tissue at the joint is also very thick. Surrounding the ossicles, which are almost the same size as in an adult, is mesen-

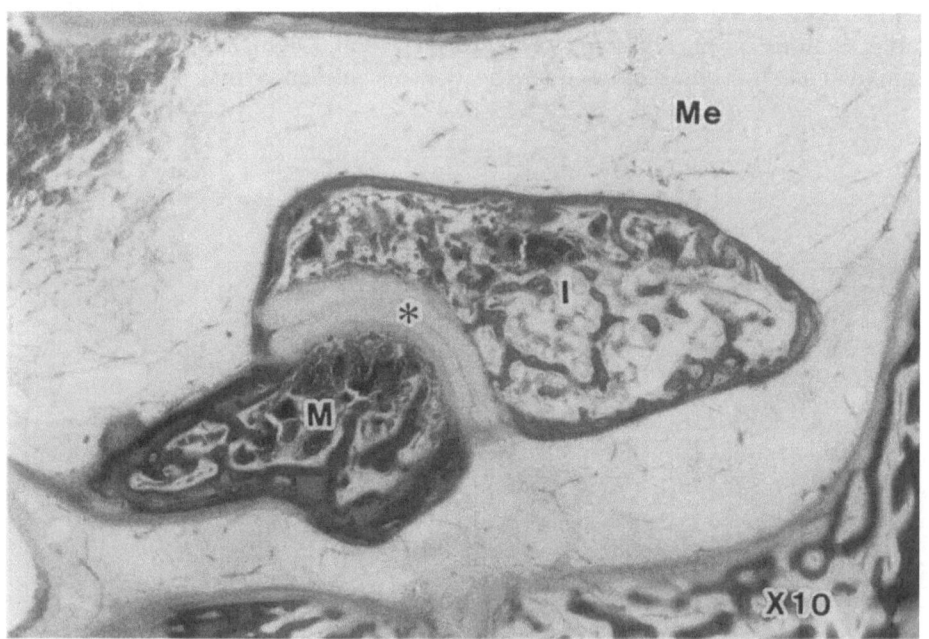

FIG. 2–12. Ossicles in the tympanic space at 5 months gestation. *M*, malleus; *I*, incus; *Me*, mesenchymal tissue around the ossicles. *Asterisk* (*) indicates cartilage at the joint

FIG. 2–13. Tympanic space at 6 months gestation. *Arrows* indicate fibrous connective tissue, the prodromal stage of mucosal folds or ligaments. *M*, malleus; *I*, incus; *Me*, mesenchymal tissue; *Ie*, internal ear canal; *Mcf*, middle cranial fossa; *Pcf*, posterior cranial fossa; *C*, cochlea; *S*, semicircular canal; *E*, external ear canal

FIG. 2–14. Tympanic cavity in the late stage of gestation. *P*, pouches; *F*, mucosal fold; *M*, malleus; *I*, incus; *Me*, mesenchymal tissue

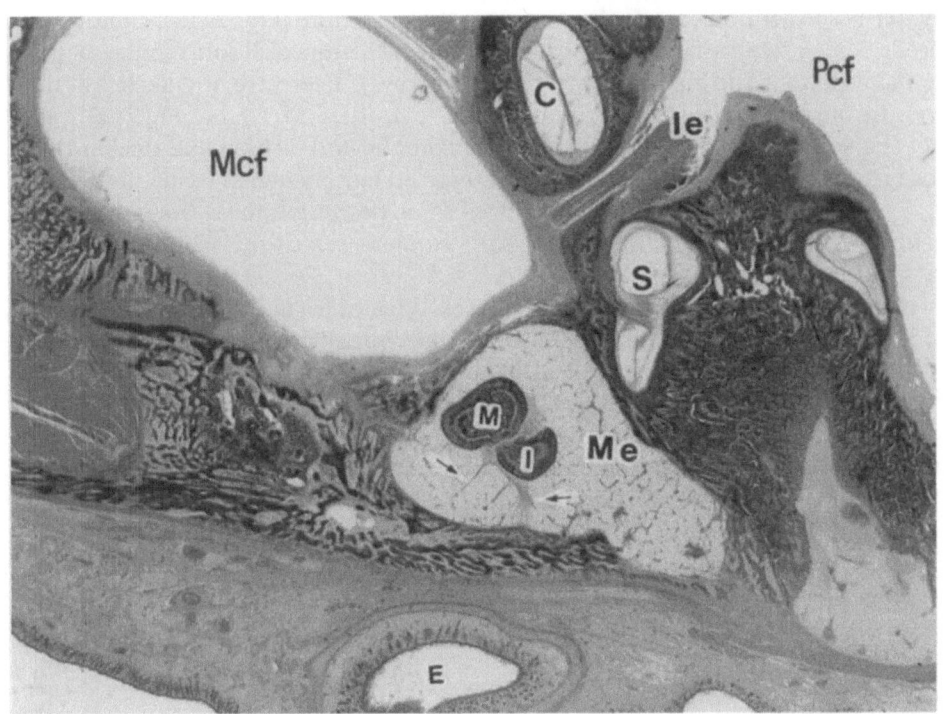

13

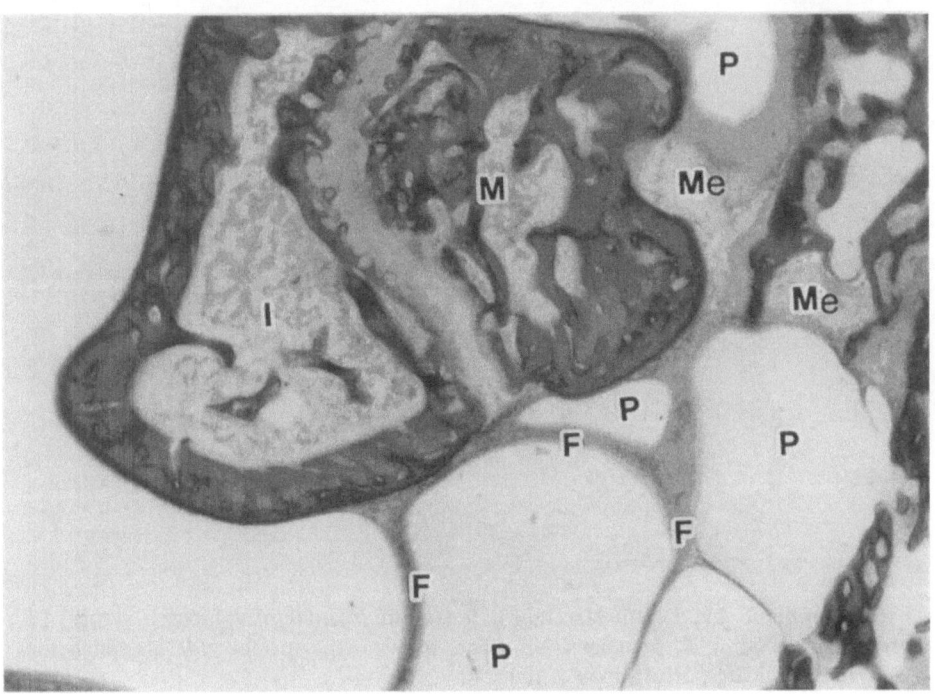

14

chymal tissue without a pouch. At 6 months gestation (Fig. 2–13), bundles of fibrous connective tissue (the prodromal stage of the mucosal folds or ligaments) are visible among the mesenchymal tissues (arrows). There are no pouches at this level. In the late stages of gestation (Fig. 2–14), there are many mucosal folds between adjoining pouches, branching in a complicated fashion and thicker than those in an adult. Among them appears scattered mesenchymal tissue. In the last stage of gestation (Fig. 2–15), the mucosal folds become thinner and very often perforated (see arrows), although the area remains relatively rich in mesenchymal tissue.

Three-dimensional reconstructions in each stage of gestation are shown in Fig. 2–16. At 3 months gestation (Fig. 2–16a), the tympanic cleft is a simple pouch reaching to the level of the malleal handle without branching, as reported by Proctor (1964). At 4 months gestation (Fig. 2–16b), the pouch fills in the hypotympanum and begins to grow upward, branching between the ossicles. It is also possible to see at this time the anterior process of the malleus (asterisk) and a bony ledge at the anterior tympanic wall (double arrows).

At 5 months gestation (Fig. 2–16c), the pouch branches into four sacks, as reported by Proctor. The saccus anticus is divided further by the tensor

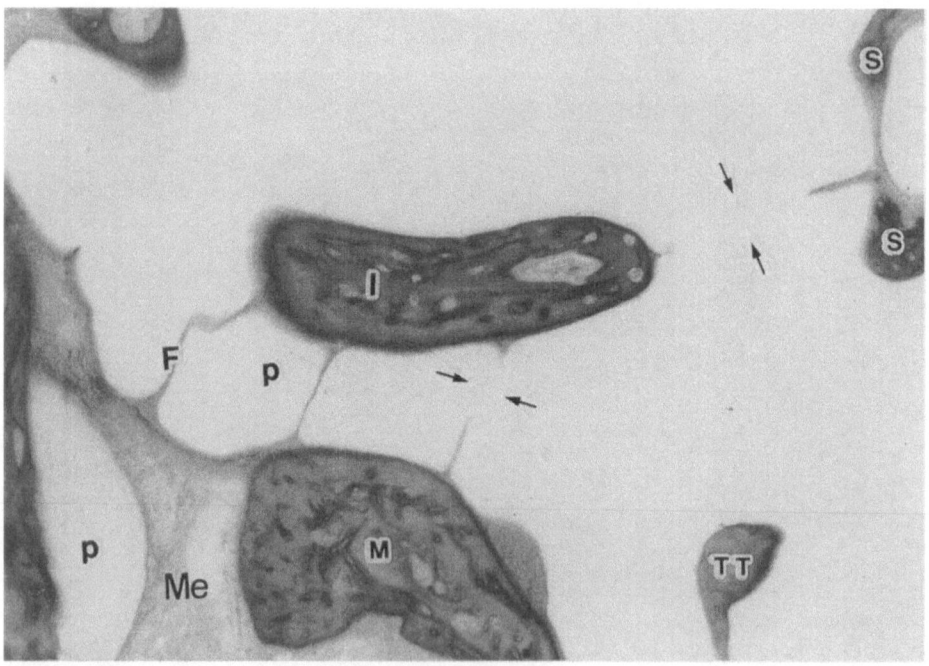

Fig. 2–15. Tympanic cavity in the last stage of gestation. *M*, malleus; *I*, incus; *S*, stapes; *TT*, tensor tympani tendon; *P*, pouches; *F*, mucosal fold, not perforated; *Me*, mesenchymal tissue. *Arrows* indicate perforations of the folds

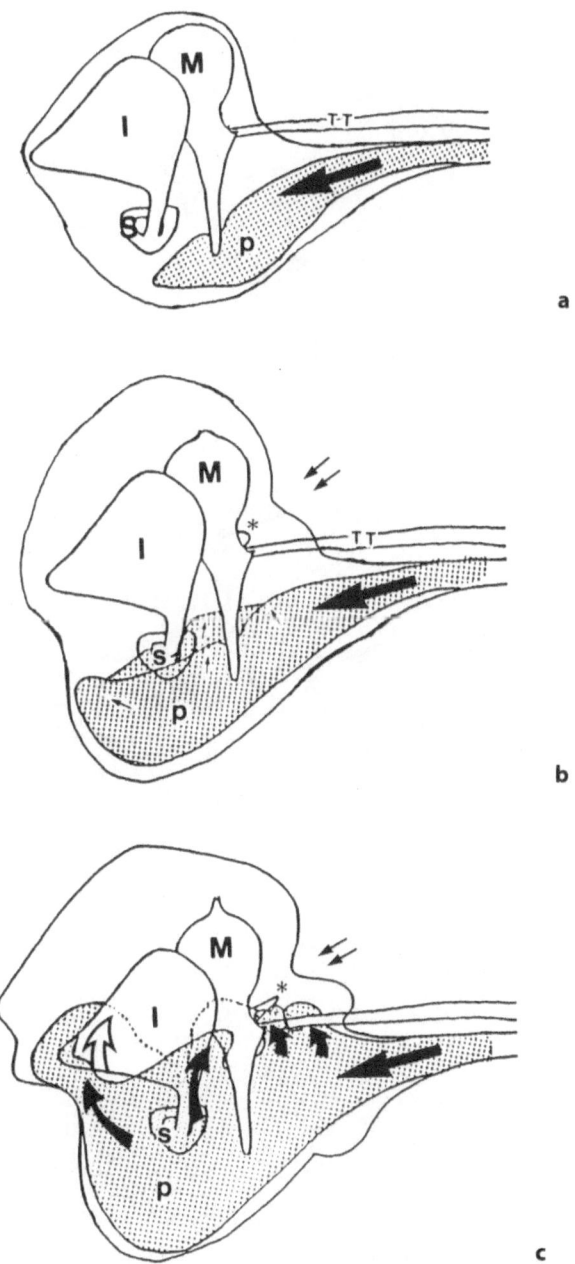

Fig. 2-16a-e. Developmental process of the tympanic space. Time of gestation: **a**, 3 months; **b**, 4 months; **c**, 5 months; **d**, 7 months; **e**, 9–10 months. *Large arrows* indicate direction of development of the pouches. *Double small arrows* indicate the bony ledge in which the supratubal recess develops after birth. *M*, malleus; *I*, incus; *S*, stapes; *P*, pouch; *TT*, tensor tympani muscle; *Pr*, Prussak's space; *asterisk*, anterior process of the malleus

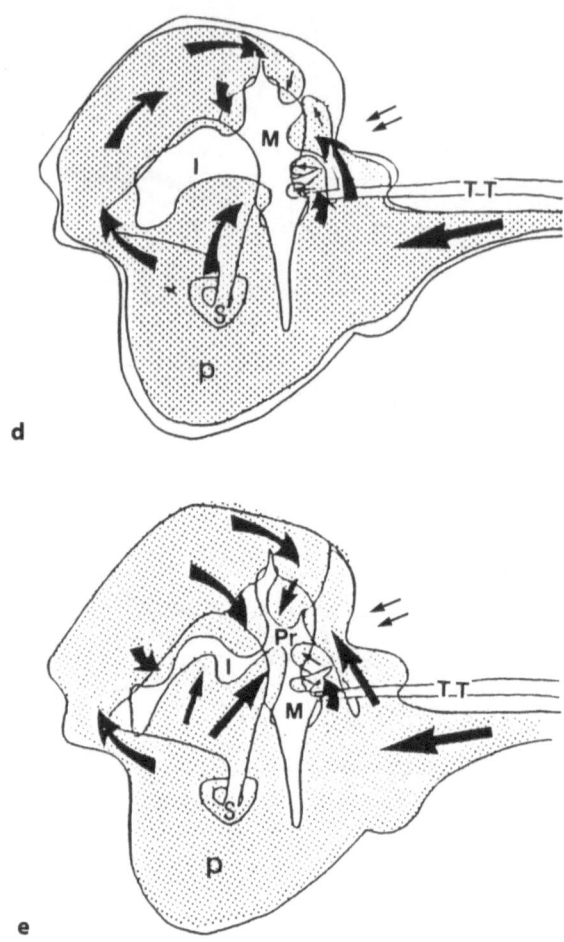

d

e

Fɪɢ. 2–16a–e. *Continued*

tympani tendon into the labyrinthine branch and the eardrum branch. Development of the latter branch stops at the lower level, and that of the former branch stops at the upper level, of the anterior process of the malleus. The branches develop later into the inferior and superior supratubal recess, respectively.

The saccus medius develops upward between the ossicles and the labyrinth, and then is divided into anterior and posterior branches by the superior mallear ligament. The former branch of the saccus medius goes down over the malleal head in the direction of the anterior process of the malleus, to make the anterior attic compartment. The saccus superior and the saccus posterior become the mastoid antrum and the retrotympanum, respectively. After 7 months gestation (Fig. 2–16d,e), four pouches begin to branch out minutely around the ossicles, being divided by the anticipated ligaments or main mucosal folds in the mesenchymal tissue and contacting each other to make the indefinite mucosal folds. The apices of both saccus medius and saccus superior develop like fingers grasping the malleal head and incudal body, to meet at Prussak's space.

Our most important finding was that there is no space in the petrous bone that coincides with the supratubal recess in the fetal middle ear cleft, as shown in Fig. 2–17a,b, which shows the view from the labyrinthine side. At the front of the malleal head, development of the saccus medius and the saccus anticus varies individually, and these do not contact each other before birth; thus a bony ledge is left between them. This bony ledge remains superior when the growth of the saccus anticus (black asterisk) is greater than that of the saccus medius (Fig. 2–17a). When growth of the saccus medius is greater than growth of the saccus anticus (white asterisk), the bony ledge remains inferior (Fig. 2–17b). We concluded that the supratubal recess could not be found in the nine fetal ears examined, and that it begins to develop gradually directly before or after birth.

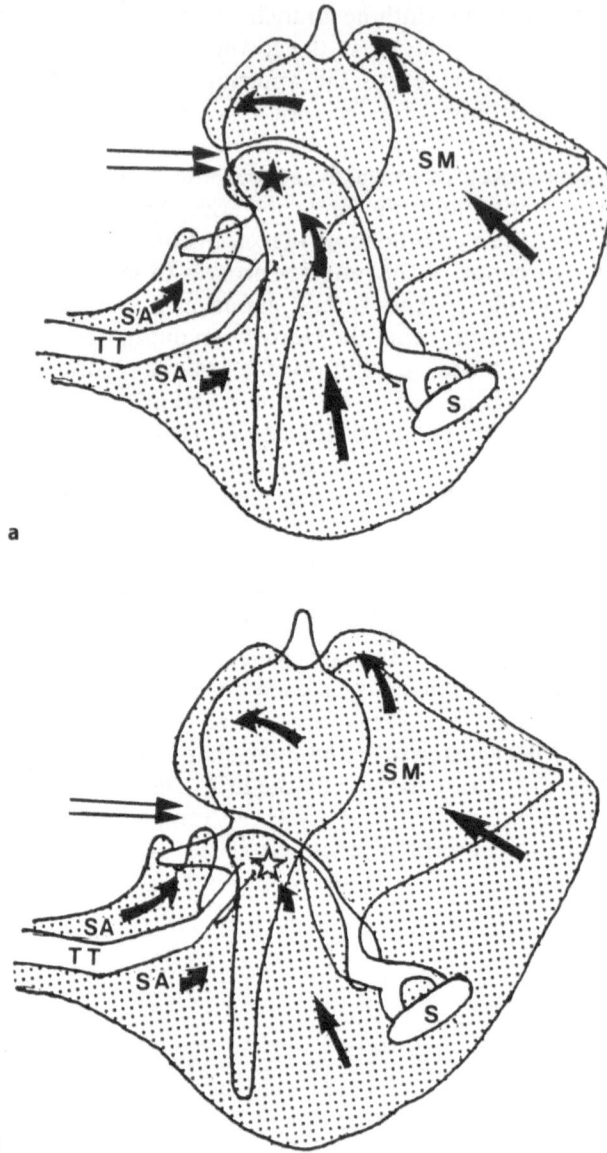

Fig. 2–17a,b. Genesis of individual differences in position of the supratubal recess, viewed from the labyrinthine side. **a** The supratubal recess will be located more superiorly if development of the saccus anticus (*black star*) dominates that of the saccus medius. *Single arrows* show the direction of the development of saccuses. *Double arrows* indicate the site of the supratubal recess. **b** The supratubal recess will be located more inferiorly if development of the saccus anticus (*white star*) is less than that of the saccus medius. *SA*, saccus anticus; *SM*, saccus medius; *TT*, tensor tympani muscle and tendon; *S*, stapes

2.3 Temporal Bone in Neonates and Children

From the collection at the Otopathology Laboratory, University of Minnesota, 92 temporal bones sectioned serially horizontally from neonates and children under 10 years of age were selected at random (Tono et al. 1996). They were divided into five groups by age: preterm newborns at 24 to 36 weeks gestation (17 bones); full-term newborns from birth to 7 days old (17 bones); infants aged 1 week to 12 months (22 bones); children 1 to 2 years old (13 bones); and children 3 to 10 years old (23 bones).

2.3.1 Mastoid Pneumatization and Age

The degree of mastoid pneumatization (PN) was classified into three categories: PN−, 42 bones with minimal formation of bony trabeculae along the mastoid antrum; PN±, 19 bones with rich bony trabeculae along the mastoid antrum; and PN+, 31 bones with mastoid air cells. Mastoid pneumatization clearly progresses with increased age (Fig. 2–18).

2.3.2 Shape of the Supratubal Recess

The shape of the supratubal recess (STR) was classified into three categories: underdeveloped STR (27 bones in which upward extension of the STR did not

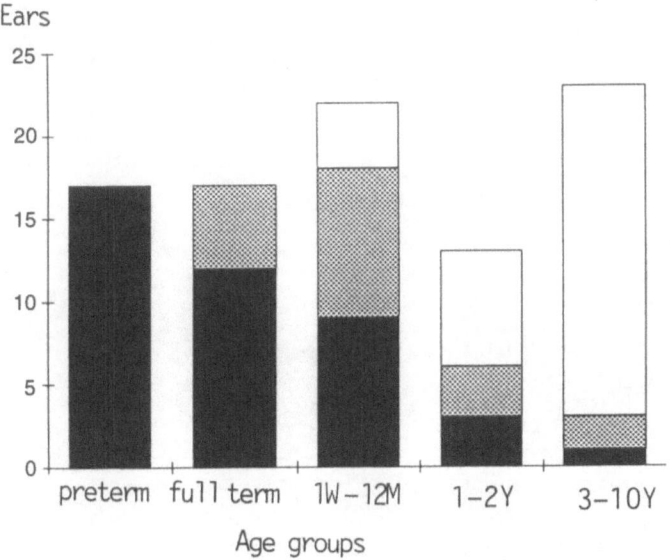

Fig. 2–18. Relationships among five age groups and their grades of pneumatization: age groups preterm, full term, 1 week–12 months, 1–2 years, or 3–10 years with grades of pneumatization − (*black bars*), ± (*stippled bars*), or + (*white bars*)

reach the level of the geniculate fossa); dome-shaped STR (57 bones with a distinct dome-shaped extension up to the level of the geniculate fossa); air cell-shaped STR (8 bones with a small STR surrounded by round or oval air cells similar in size). Figure 2–19a shows an air cell-shaped STR and Fig. 2–19b a dome-shaped STR.

Incidences of these STR shapes by age groups and by degree of pneumatization are shown in Figs. 2–20 and 2–21, respectively. In the latest fetal stage, the eustachian tube (saccus anticus) begins to expand upward and reaches the level of the geniculate fossa, forming a dome-like STR, in most cases by the end of the first year after birth.

Air cell-shaped STRs are always found in children more than 3 years old who have well-pneumatized mastoids and occur about one-third as often as dome-shaped STRs. The STR cannot be recognized in 60% of all poorly pneumatized ears; other poorly pneumatized ears have a dome-shaped STR. Of well-pneumatized ears, on the other hand, three-fourths have a dome-shaped STR and one-fourth have an air cell-shaped STR. We concluded that the STR develops at first as a dome-shaped space until 3 years of age, and then air cells develop around the STR in parallel with pneumatization.

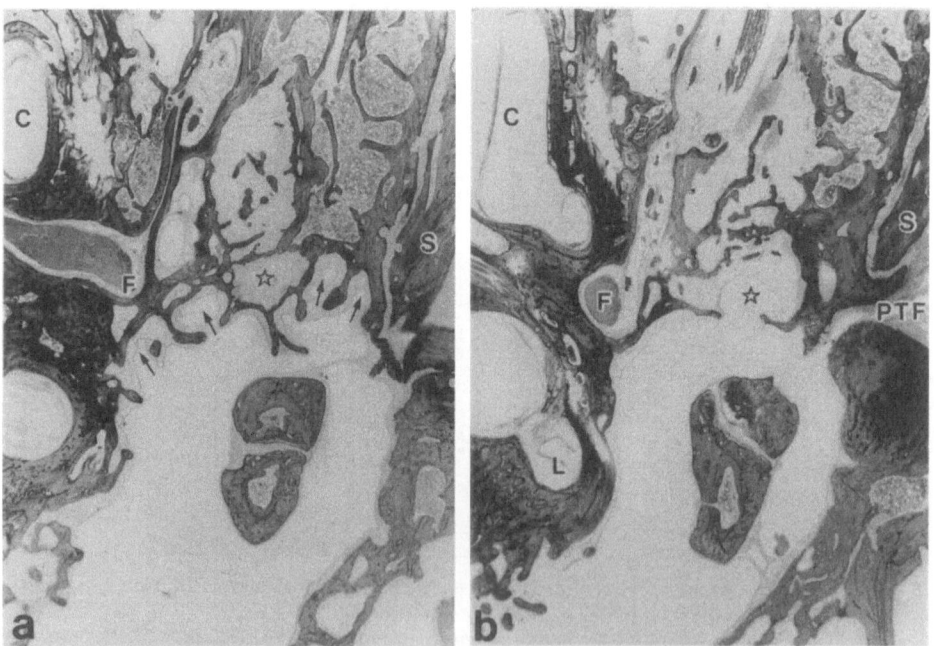

Fig. 2–19a,b. Shapes of the supratubal recess (STR). **a** Air cell-shaped STR (*star*). **b** Dome-shaped STR (*star*). *Arrows*, air cells. *F*, facial nerve; *C*, cochlea; *PTF*, petro-tympanal fissure; *S*, squamosa; *L*, labyrinth

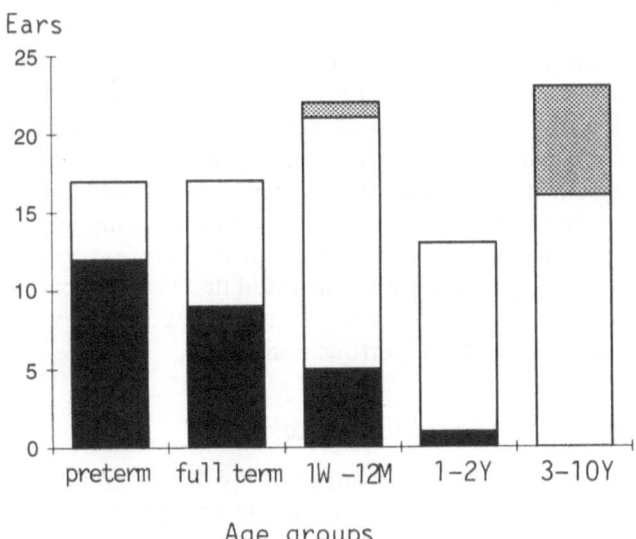

Fig. 2–20. Incidence of three types of STR [underdeveloped (*black bars*), dome shaped (*white bars*), or air cell shaped (*stippled bars*)] in five age groups: preterm, full term, 1 week–12 months, 1–2 years, or 3–10 years

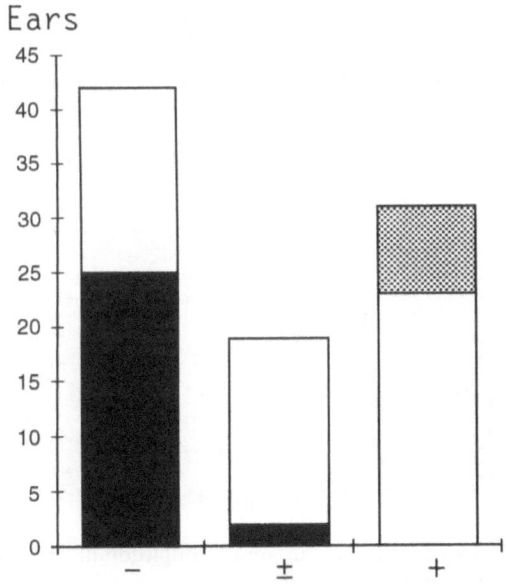

Fig. 2–21. Incidence of STRs [underdeveloped (*black bars*), dome shaped (*white bars*), or air cell shaped (*stippled bars*)] by degree of pneumatization [(−), (±), or (+)]

2.3.3 Size of the Supratubal Recess

Using 57 sections from dome-shaped STRs cut at the level of the geniculate fossa, the maximum longitudinal width (1) and the maximum transverse width (2) of the STR as well as the transverse width of the anterior petrosal tegmen (3) were measured, as shown in Fig. 2–22. The charts in Fig. 2–23 show mean values of these measurements, plotted against age groups and against degree of pneumatization. The STR tends to enlarge with increasing age as well as with progression of pneumatization. As the width of the anterior petrosal tegmen was found to be relatively constant, it was suggested that active expansion of the STR in the anterior petrous tegmen is more important than its passive enlargement as the result of enlargement of the petrous bone itself.

2.3.4 Contents of the Supratubal Recess

The contents of the STR, by age groups and by degree of pneumatization, are shown in Fig. 2–24. In the STR, decrease in mesenchymal tissue and increase in aerated space proceed in step with progress of age and degree of pneumatization. (In this study, the incidence of scars from probable otitis media also showed a tendency to increase in the air space.)

2.3.5 Patterns of Communication with the Supratubal Recess

Patterns of communication of the STR with surrounding spaces at the level of the geniculate fossa were studied in specimens of temporal bone (Fig. 2–25). In Fig. 2–25a, the STR is separated from the epitympanum by a bony wall (arrow) and

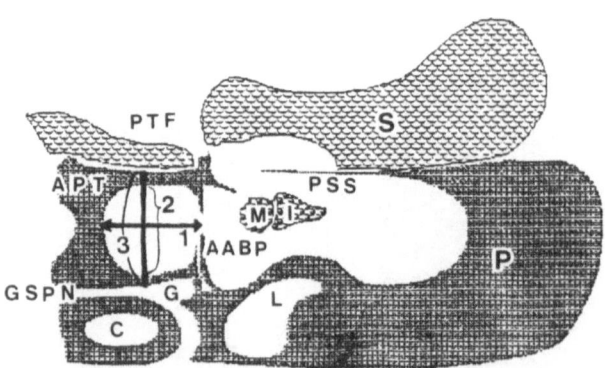

Fig. 2–22. Measurements of STRs. *1*, maximum longitudinal width of STR; *2*, maximum transverse width of STR; *3*, transverse width of the anterior petrosal tegmen. *AABP*, anterior attic bony plate; *APT*, anterior petrosal tegmen; *GSPN*, greater superficial petrosal nerve; *G*, geniculate ganaglion; *PTF*, petrotympanic fissura; *PSS*, petrosquamous suture; *P*, petrosa; *S*, squamosa; *M*, malleus; *I*, incus; *C*, cochlea; *L*, lateral semicircular canal

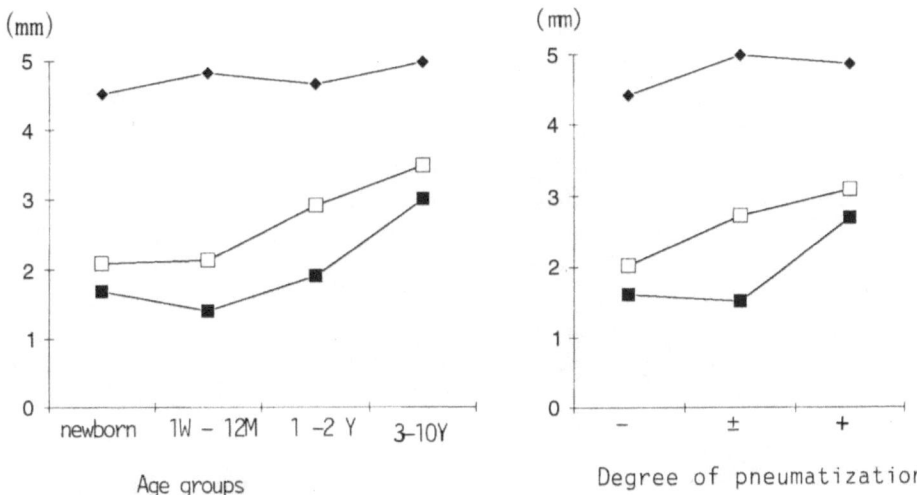

Fig. 2–23. Sizes of STRs by age groups (*left*) and degree of penumatization (*right*). *Black squares*, width of anterior petrosal tegmen (APT); *white squares*, width of STR; *diamonds*, length of STR

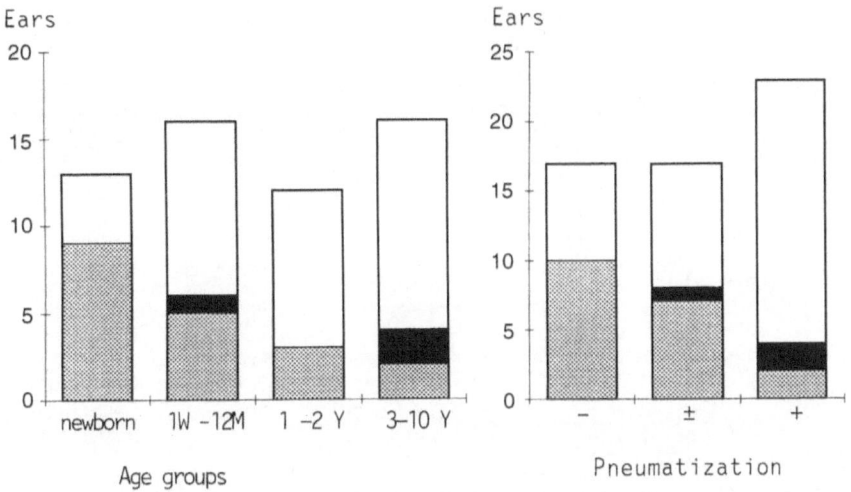

Fig. 2–24. Contents of STRs by age groups (*left*) and pneumatization (*right*). *White bars*, air; *black bars*, scar; *stippled bars*, mesenchyme

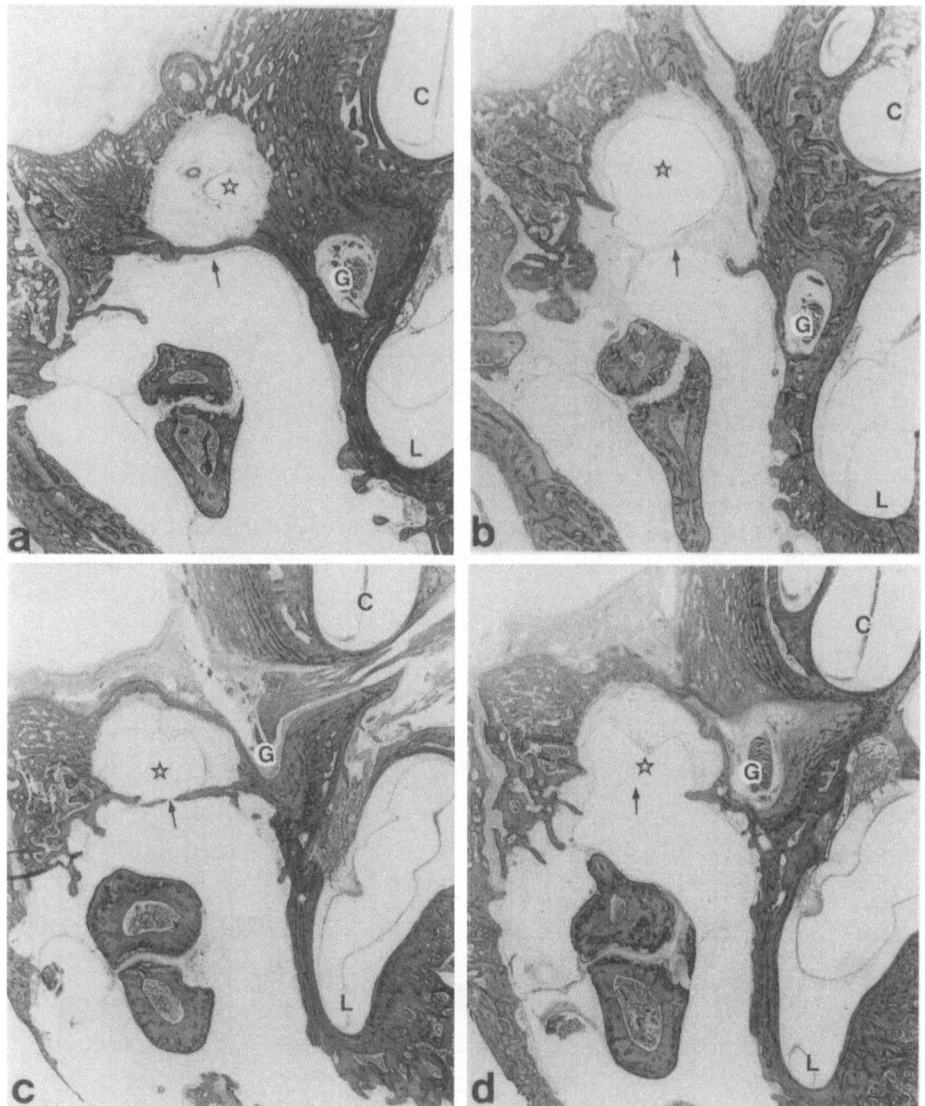

Fɪɢ. 2–25a–d. Communication of STR with surrounding spaces. **a** STR (*star*) is separated by bony wall (*arrow*) from the epitympanum. **b** STR (*star*) is separated by mucosal fold (*arrow*) from the epitympanum. **c** STR (*star*) communicates through small bony defect (*arrow*). **d** STR (*star*) communicates through large defect of mucosal fold (*arrow*). *G*, facial nerve or geniculate ganglion; *C*, cochlea; *L*, lateral semicircular canal

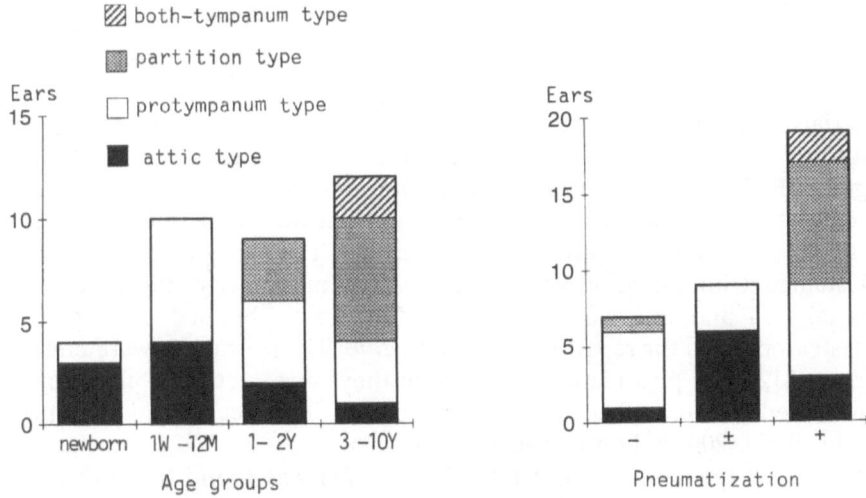

Fig. 2–26. Patterns of communication of STR with surrounding spaces by age (*left*) and pneumatization (*right*)

is rich in mesenchymal tissue, with a small aerated space (asterisk). In Fig. 2–25b, the STR is separated by a mucosal fold (arrow) from the epitympanum. Both STRs communicate only with the protympanum. On the other hand, the STRs in Fig. 2–25c,d are in direct communication with the epitympanum through the incomplete bony (Fig. 2–25c) or mucosal (Fig. 2–25d) partition.

Patterns of communication of the STR were studied in serial sections, observing upward and downward from the recess. Patterns could be classified as follows: (1) an STR with an aerated space communicating only with the epitympanum (attic type); (2) an STR communicating only with the protympanum (protympanic type); (3) an STR with a membranous and/or bony partition dividing it into two portions, the anterior communicating with the protympanum and the posterior with the epitympanum (partitioned type); and (4) an STR without partition, communicating with the pro- and epitympanum (both-tympanums type).

Incidence of these types, by age group and by degree of pneumatization, is shown in Fig. 2–26. Aeration of the STR comes initially from either the protympanum or the attic in early infancy. The partitioned type of STR appears only after 1 year of age and is increasingly found in older age groups, indicating that this type is formed with postnatal growth of the temporal bone. The both-tympanums type appears only in the group 3 to 10 years of age or in the group with well-pneumatized STRs, indicating that this type shows the last stage of development of the STR.

2.4 Fine Structure of Mucosal Folds and Mucosa

2.4.1 Normal Mucosal Fold

Materials for light microscopic study were obtained from normal temporal bones at autopsy (Morimitsu 1991). The temporal bones were fixed with a 3% solution of glutaraldehyde. The tensor tympani and anterior attic mucosal folds were removed under a binocular microscope and then were embedded in Epok 812 (Kohken, Tokyo) after fixation with osmic acid. The specimens were sectioned and stained with toluidine blue. For electron microscopy, the anterior attic mucosal fold and the superior mallear fold were obtained at surgeries for cholesteatoma and for repair of the facial nerve. The specimens were embedded in Epon 812 after postfixation in osmium; they were sectioned ultrathinly and then stained with uranyl acetate and lead citrate. The electron microscope used was the JEOL 200 (Nihon Densi, Tokyo).

The tensor tympani mucosal fold (Fig. 2–27a) was found to be three times thicker than the anterior attic mucosal fold (Fig. 2–27b). Its lamina propria consisted of richly collagenous fiber mixed with elastic fibers. Therefore, it is considered possible that the tensor tympani mucosal fold may become a strong partition against which negative pressure may cause retraction cholesteatomas in the attic, if the mucosa is not perforated. On the other hand, the lamina propria of the anterior attic mucosal fold (Fig. 2–27b) has loose connective tissue without elastic fibers. Both mucosal folds have simple squamous epithelium and capillaries. Corpuscles (including nerve fibers like Pacchionian bodies, reported by Lim 1975) were, however, not found in our materials.

The superior mallear fold (Fig. 2–27c) was covered with simple squamous epithelium with microvilli. Its lamina propria consisted of pseudo-stratified fibrocysts with loose collagenous fibers. In this fold were found scattered amyelinated nerve fibers (Fig. 2–27d), thought to be free axon ending, although neither mitochondria nor secretory granules were present. The blood vessels (Fig. 2–27e) had nonfenestrated endothelium and were partially covered with pericytes.

2.4.2 Pathological Mucosal Fold

Figure 2–28 presents mucosal folds in contact with the perimatrix of cholesteatoma. In the perimatrix (Fig. 2–28a), there are pseudo-stratified columnar epithelium and infiltration of inflammatory cells; foreign-body macrophages are seen around cholesterin crystals (Fig. 2–28b). Among the mucosal cells left in granulation tissue, there are columnar cells with secretory granules (Fig. 2–28c). These findings coincide with those in Wullstein's (1976) report on the mucosal folds found in chronic otitis media. Furthermore, there are young vessels with narrow lumens in the granulation tissue (Fig. 2–28d). This finding seems to indicate the active correspondence of granulation tissue to vigorous metabolism.

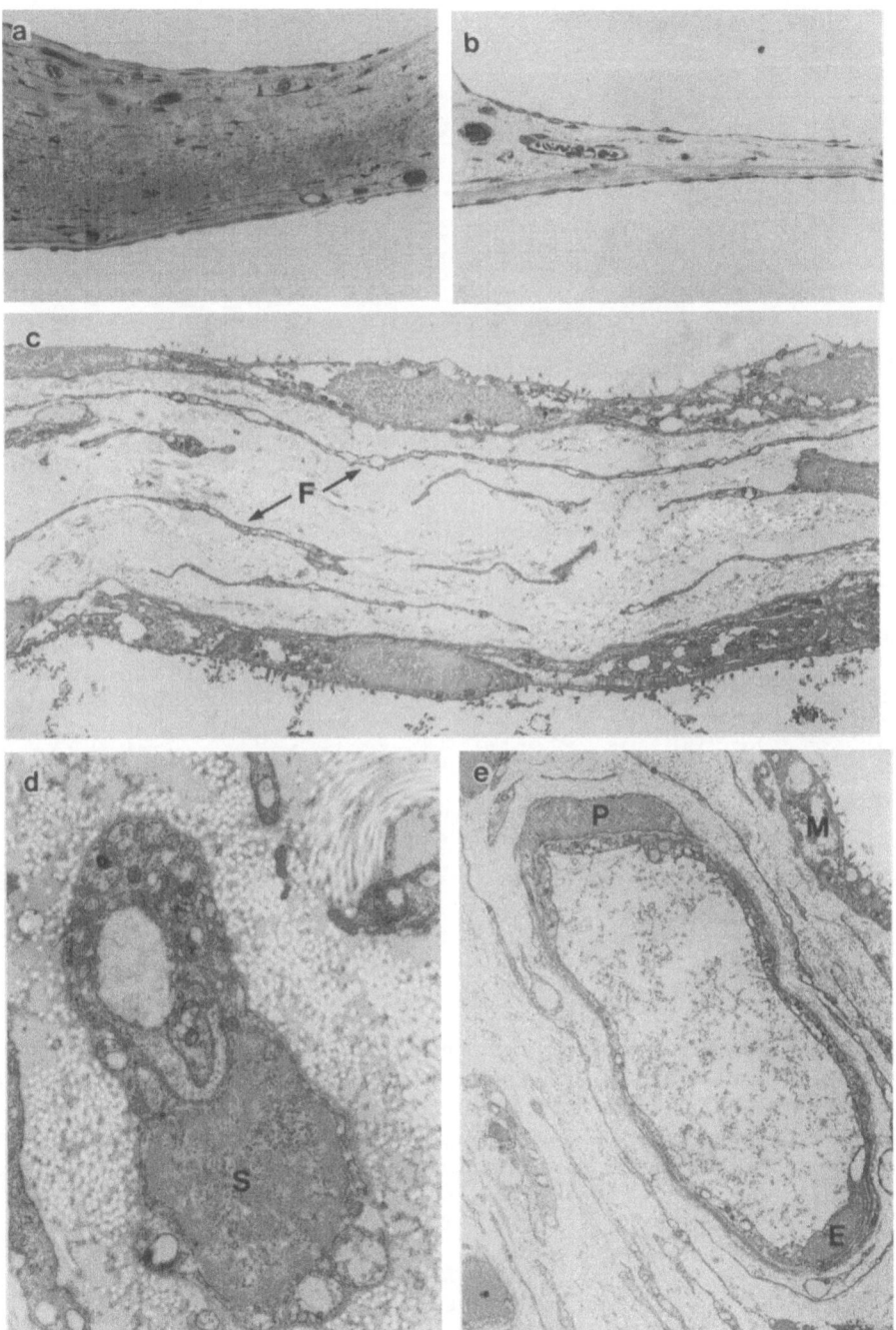

Fɪɢ. 2–27a–e. Fine structure of normal mucosal folds. **a** Tensor tympani mucosal fold (light microscopy, ×290). **b** Anterior attic mucosal fold (light microscopy, ×300). **c** Superior mallear fold (electron microscopy, ×4500). *F*, fibrocytes. **d** Amyelinated nerve fiber in mallear fold (electron microscopy, ×13000). *S*, Schwann's cell. **e** Blood vessel in mallear fold (electron microscopy, ×32000). *P*, pericyte; *E*, endothelium; *M*, mucosal folds

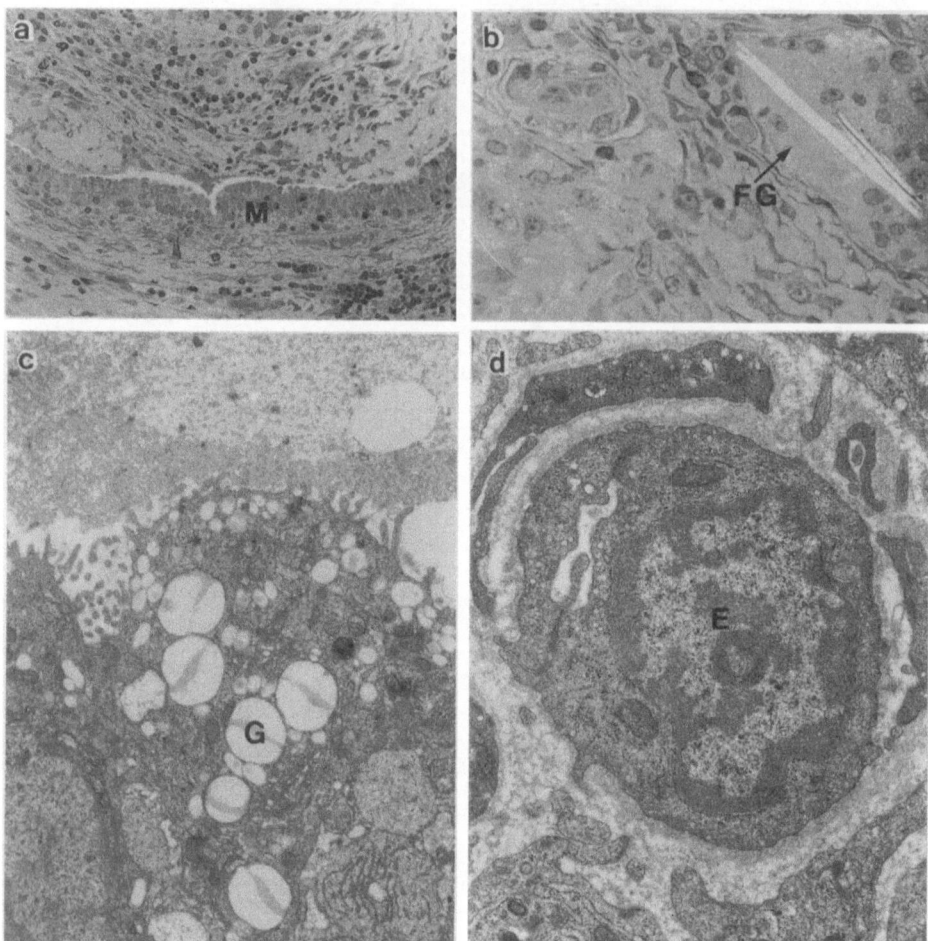

Fɪɢ. 2–28a–d. Fine structure of pathological mucosal folds. **a** Perimatrix of cholesteatoma (light microscopy, ×500). *M*, columnar epithelium. **b** Foreign-body macrophage at cholesterin crystal (light microscopy, ×920). *FG*, foreign-body macrophage. **c** Columnar cell with secretory granules (electron microscopy, ×90000). *G*, secretory granule. **d** Young vessel in granulation tissue. *E*, endothelium

From the findings observed, we believe the mucosal fold becomes hypertrophic and thick and its epithelium changes to pseudo-stratified, gaining a secretory function when the fold comes into contact with the perimatrix of cholesteatoma. There are opposing opinions as to whether the mucosal fold plays a role as a protective barrier against the growth of cholesteatoma. So far as we can see, the normal mucosal fold is so thin (and often perforated) that is would not be very useful as a barrier. The fold changes, however, to a thicker one in pathological

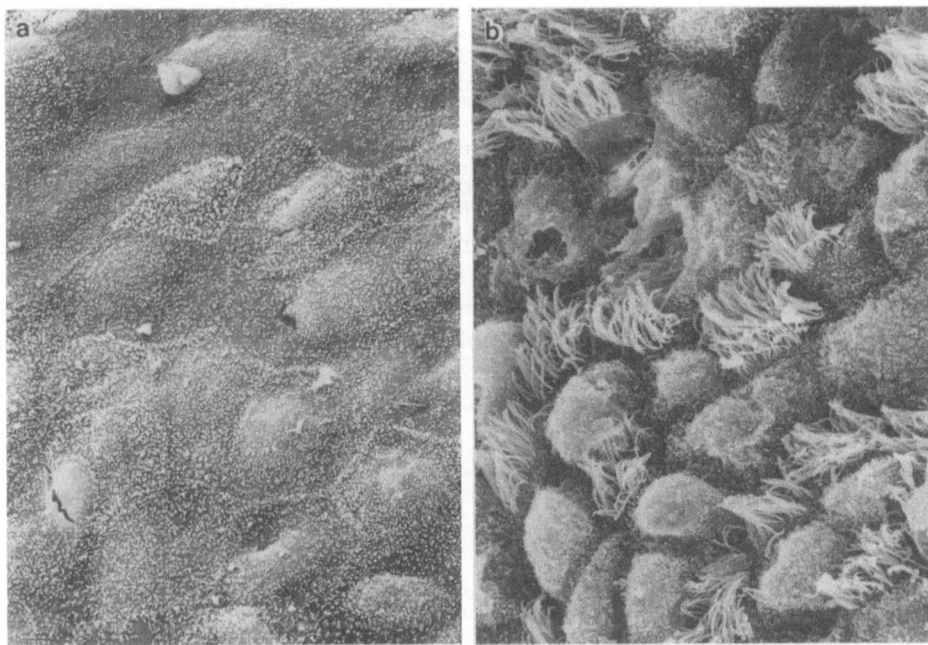

Fɪɢ. 2–29a,b. Superficial structure of mucosa. **a** Mucosa of the anterior attic mucosal fold (scanning electron microscopy, ×3000). **b** Mucosa of the supratubal recess (scanning electron microscopy, ×2700)

conditions like those observed here, so it may be possible that it then can act as a protective barrier against the growth of cholesteatoma in some pathological conditions.

2.4.3 Superficial Structure of Mucosa

The superficial structures of the mucosa and mucosal fold were studied using a scanning electron microscope (Fig. 2–29) and reported in 1991 by Morimitsu. The epithelium of the anterior attic mucosal fold was found to be polymorphic and squamous with microvilli and also with ciliated epithelium (Fig. 2–29a). Epithelium at the supratubal recess, on the other hand, was mucoepithelium with microvilli, showing a scattering of ciliated epithelium (Fig. 2–29b). Concerning distribution of ciliated epithelium in the tympanic cavity, Shimada and Lim (1972) reported that ciliated cells increase from the epitympanum to the eustachian tube. Hoshino (1990) also observed ciliated epithelium in the supratubal recess. We conclude that new ventilation routes made in anterior tympanotomy may also have some transportive function as they are covered with ciliated epithelium.

2.5 Developmental Processes of the Supratubal Recess

Developmental processes of the STR in a normally pneumatized ear are illustrated in Fig. 2–30. Our study showed that upward expansion of the osseous eustachian tube (saccus anticus) into the petrous bone begins at the latest stage of gestation. The saccus is divided by the tensor tympani tendon into two branches, the labyrinthine branch and the tympanic branch. The former continues to expand throughout childhood, forming the superior STR; the latter stays in position, making the inferior STR.

These observations are supported by results obtained in examinations of adult temporal bone; i.e., that the correlation between the size of the STR and the grade of pneumatization is proportional for the superior STR but inverse for the inferior STR. Therefore it is possible to say that the STR is a cavity that differs

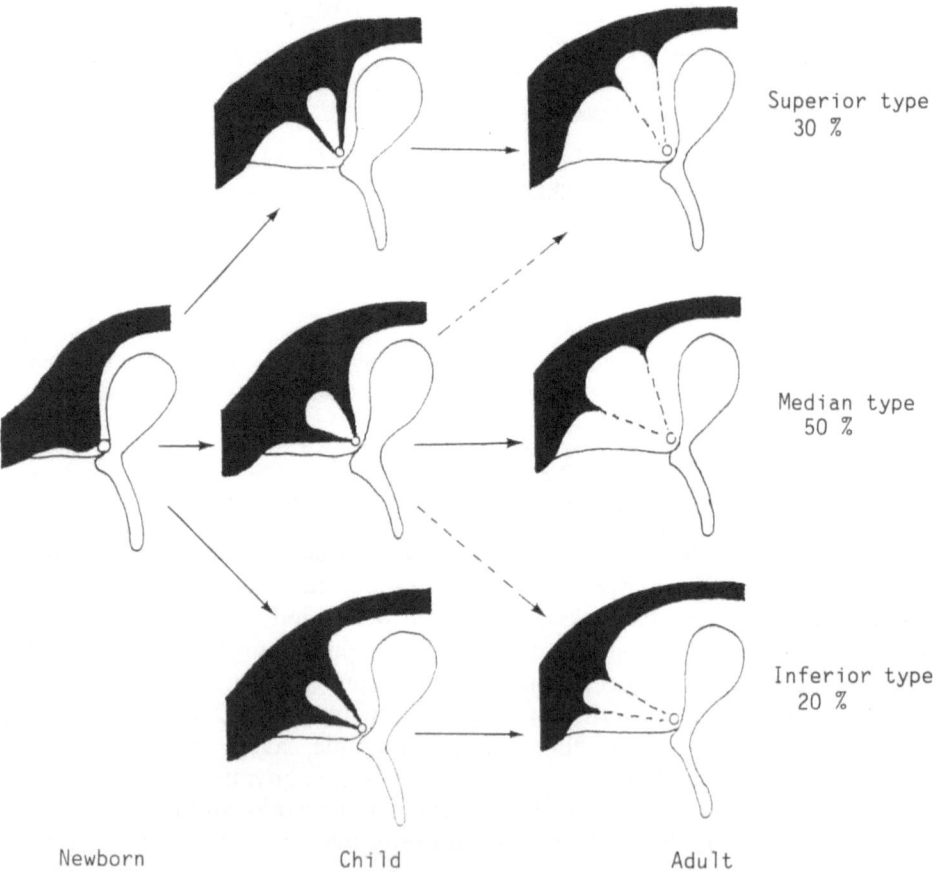

Superior type
30 %

Median type
50 %

Inferior type
20 %

Newborn   Child   Adult

FIG. 2–30. Developmental process of the supratubal recess in the normal ear

from the tympanic cavities and the mastoid antrum, which virtually complete their expansion by the end of gestation.

The osseous eustachian tube elongates after birth in proportion to the forward shift of the anterior petrosal tegmen because of growth, creating a space for the STR anterior to the protympanum. Further anterior growth of the petrosal tegmen is apparently achieved by pneumatization of the petrous bone and peritubal cells or by the expansion of the STR itself. If development of the saccus anticus is greater or more rapid than development of the saccus medius, the STR locates more superiorly. This type, found in 30% of all STRs, is called the superior type of STR. In 20% of all ears, the STR locates more inferiorly; these are called the inferior type of STR. In 50% of ears we examined, the STR was located medially; here it is called the median type of STR. Of course, many ears are difficult to classify into these three types because of variations among the types.

The superior STR is aerated by the labyrinthine branch of the saccus anticus. This space, therefore, is assumed not be included embryologically in the epitympanum but rather in the protympanum. The anterior attic bony plate becomes shorter, changing into the anterior attic mucosal fold, which becomes even thinner, perforates, and then disappears. The tensor tympani bony plate and its mucosal fold also show the same progress, although their levels of disappearance are different individually. The STR communicates to either the protympanum or the epitympanum in childhood and then to both cavities as pneumatization progresses. Thus the anterior part of the tympanic diaphragm comes to be perforated, ventilating through the STR into the epitympanum, as well as through the tympanic isthmus in normally pneumatized ears.

We concluded that formation of the STR is independent of formation of the other tympanic cavities, and that it relates more to the degree and nature of pneumatization of the temporal bone.

References

Ars B (1986) The morphogenesis of the tympani part of the temporal bone. Clin Otolaryngol (Oxf) 11:9–13

Chatellier HP, Lemoine J (1946) Le diaphragme interattico-tympanique du nouveau-ne. Ann d'Oto-Laryngol 13:534–566

Declau F (1989) Normal growth patterns of the middle ear cleft in the human fetus. J Laryngol Otol 103:461–465

Gacek RR (1980) Surgical landmark for the facial nerve in the epitympanum. Ann Otol Rhinol Laryngol 89:249–250

Horn KL, Brackmann DE, Luxford WM, Shea JJ (1986) The supratubal recess in cholesteatoma surgery. Ann Otol Rhinol Laryngol 95:12–15

Hoshino T (1988) Surgical anatomy of the anterior epitympanic space. Arch Otolaryngol Head Neck Surg 114:1143–1145

Hoshino T (1990) Observation of the epithelium in the supratubal recess with a scanning electron microscope. Clin Otol Jpn 17:50–51

Hoshino T, Suzuki J (1978) Anterior attic wall anatomy. Arch Otolaryngol 104:588–590

Lim D (1975) Human middle ear corpuscles: a light- and electron-microscopic study. Laryngoscope 85:1725–1737

Morimitsu T (1991) Etiology of middle ear cholesteatoma. Otol Fukuoka 37(Suppl 1):271–405

Proctor B (1964) The development of the middle ear spaces and their surgical significance. J Laryngol Otol 78:631–648

Proctor B (1989) Surgical anatomy of the ear. Blackwell, Oxford

Schuknecht HF, Gulya AJ (1986) Anatomy of the temporal bone with surgical implications. Lea and Febiger, Philadelphia, p 89

Sheehy JL (1979) Otolaryngology. Harper and Row, Hagerstown, p 67

Shimada T, Lim D (1972) Distribution of ciliated cells in the human middle ear. Ann Otol Rhinol Laryngol 81:203–211

Shimizu S (1987) Embryological study on middle ear cavity in the human fetus (In Japanese with English abstract). Oto-Rhino-Laryngol (Tokyo) 30:155–175

Tono T, Schachern PA, Morizono T, Paparella MM, Morimitsu T (1996) Developmental anatomy of the supratubal recess in temporal bones from fetuses and children. Am J Otol 17:99–107

Wigand ME, Trillsch K (1974) Surgical anatomy of the sinus epitympani. Ann Otol Rhinol Laryngol 82:378–382

Wullstein SR (1976) Histopathological alternations of the mucosal folds in chronic otitis media. Acta Otolaryngol (Stockholm) 81:197–199

Wullstein SR (1984) The epitympanum and ossicular chain. In: Marquet JFE (ed) Surgery and pathology of middle ear. Nijhoff, Boston, pp 61–64

Chapter 3
Anterior Tympanotomy:
A Surgical Technique for Cholesteatoma

3.1 Historical Considerations and Naming of Anterior Tympanotomy

Surgery for cholesteatoma began with radical operations and then conservative radical operations were developed. After proposal of the so-called canal-up technique for chronic otitis media in the 1960s, this technique was used with great expectations even for cholesteatoma. In particular, Jansen's (1967) posterior tympanotomy technique and Sheehy's "intact canal wall" technique (Sheehy and Patterson 1967) have tended to the so-called canal-up or "closed" techniques. During the latter half of the 1970s, however, an increasing number of adverse reports began to appear that revealed alarmingly high incidences of both recurrent and residual cholesteatoma. Thus, many improved techniques were presented such as the mastoid obliteration technique (Palva 1973), the combined approach tympanoplasty (Smyth 1976; Sadé 1982), osteoplastic epitympanotomy (Wullstein 1974), the canal-down with reconstruction technique (Suzuki, 1982), the lateral tympanotomy technique (Tos 1982; Bhide 1982), and so on. No reliable technique has been reported, however, that makes use of a canal-up method in an operative procedure for cholesteatoma for general use by otologic surgeons.

Anterior tympanotomy can appear under other names. Farrier (1968) proposed the name anterior attico-tympanotomy; his was an approach to the posterior tympanic cavity from the external ear canal, not from the mastoid as in Jansen's technique. Portmann (1985) used the name superior and anterior tympanotomy, stating that this procedure opens the front of the attic and allows a view of the incudal body and the whole of the malleal head. He used this name, therefore, for the surgical procedure of opening the anterior part of the epitympanum, but not for the supratubal recess or removing the anterior attic bony plate.

There are also analogous techniques with different names. Proctor (1989) suggested a procedure to get a wide communicating route to the protympanum by removing the superior mallear fold and the tensor tympani mucosal fold. He named this technique posterior atticotomy, although no bony plates are removed. Jansen (1984) reported a surgical procedure called posterior tubotomy that opens the supratubal recess over the ossicles after an intact canal wall mastoidectomy, as in my anterior tympanotomy. Zini et al. (1989) reported a "superior tubotomy" in which the tympanic ostium of the eustachian tube is opened to the supratubal recess and opened further to the anterior part of the epitympanum by an anteriorly enlarged transmeatal atticotomy. The site they operate on in their tubotomy is, however, not the tuba auditiva but the supratubal recess belonging to the protympanum.

Naming surgical procedures is very difficult and often leads to confusion. I think the simplest method of naming is by the name of the place opened in that surgical procedure; for instance, mastoidotomy opens the mastoid cavity, tympanotomy opens the tympanic cavity, and anterior tympanotomy opens the anterior tympanic cavity (protympanum). Anterior tympanotomy is a surgical technique used always in combination with intact canal wall mastoidectomy in surgery for cholesteatoma. It was not originally a technique for eradication of the cholesteatoma matrix membrane but rather for improvement of intratympanic ventilation from the eustachian tube.

3.2 Surgical Technique in Anterior Tympanotomy Using the Canal-Up Method

3.2.1 Incision in the Skin

A retroauricular incision is made in the skin, elongating it 1.0 cm toward the preauricular helical crus (Fig. 3–1, large arrow). The upper two-thirds of the auricle is detached anteriorly and inferiorly at the layer close to the auricular perichondrium. Then a large triangular flap (Palva's flap, P) is detached from the planum mastoideum, together with its periosteum, to the zygomatic root (Z) and passing over the external ear canal. It is especially important to expose the zygomatic root (Fig. 3–1).

3.2.2 Detachment of the Skin of the Ear Canal

Under an operating microscope, skin in the left ear is detached from the bony canal wall posteriorly to 4 o'clock and anteriorly to 9 o'clock. Using fine elevators, the upper half of the eardrum is detached from the mallear handle in continuity with the skin of the canal. The skin at the introitus of its retraction (small arrow, Fig. 3–1) from the flaccid portion of the posterior superior quadrant of the eardrum is detached from the bony wall, but not removed, in this stage.

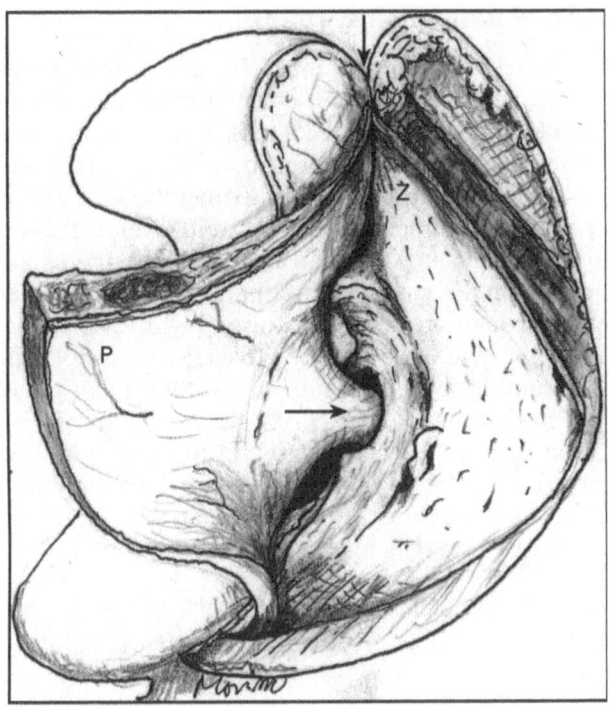

Fig. 3–1. Incision in the skin and exposure of the zygomatic root. *Large arrow*, preauricular skin incision; *small arrow*, introitus of retraction pocket. *Z*, zygomatic root; *P*, Palva's flap

3.2.3 Position of the Head in Mastoidectomy

Intact canal wall mastoidectomy is performed using cutting burrs under an operating microscope and starting from Macewen's triangle. Drilling to the mastoid antrum may be troublesome in poorly pneumatized ears with a small cholesteatoma. The superior canal wall must be thinned to the epitympanum from the mastoid side, not from the ear canal side. The exposed dura of the tegmen is a useful guide to the antrum.

After the cholesteatoma is exposed, a diamond burr is recommended for use in complete removal of the matrix membrane. Drilling must be extended anteriorly toward the zygomatic root over the ossicles, taking care to make a space in front of the malleal head. The visual axis (A) must be on the same plane as the vertical axis of the external ear canal (Fig. 3–2). With the head in this position, the anterior surface of the malleal head and the anterior attic bony plate are directly visible. With the patient's head rotated more anteriorly (B), it is impossible to see the anterior malleal head so as to eradicate the matrix membrane, and also difficult to perform anterior tympanotomy completely and keep the ossicular chain in position.

3.2.4 Eradication of Pathological Tissue

Removal of the matrix membrane must be performed while keeping the cholesteatomatous sack as intact as possible, turning the skin of the diseased matrix inside out just as one would turn a sock inside out from the tip of its toe (Fig. 3–3). A cotton ball (C) is useful to scrub off the matrix membrane, even on a blue line with no rupture of the labyrinthine membrane.

Attic cholesteatomas develop into the mastoid over the ossicular chain. In cases of tubal dysfunction, they develop into the mesotympanum through the tympanic isthmus under the ossicles. The matrical sack is pushed out into the external ear canal through an attic retraction (Fig. 3–3a). Almost all cases of adhesive cholesteatoma (Fig. 3–3b) develop from the posterior superior quadrant of an adhered eardrum through the tympanic isthmus under the ossicles. Therefore, for adhesive cholesteatomas, posterior tympanotomy (P) is usually necessary for eradication of diseased matrix around the stapes and in the tympanic sinus. After removal of the cholesteatomatous matrix, a bony wall is exposed in front of the malleal head. This bony wall (asterisk) is the anterior attic bony plate, called the anterior buttress, crista anterior, or cog.

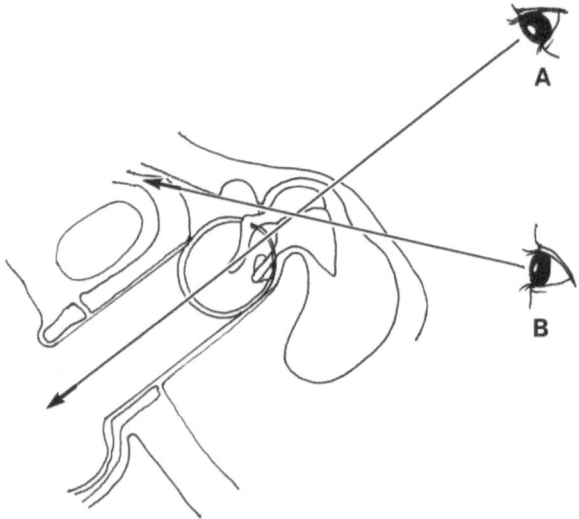

Fig. 3–2. Visual axis for anterior tympanotomy. A, optimum visual line; B, inconvenient visual line

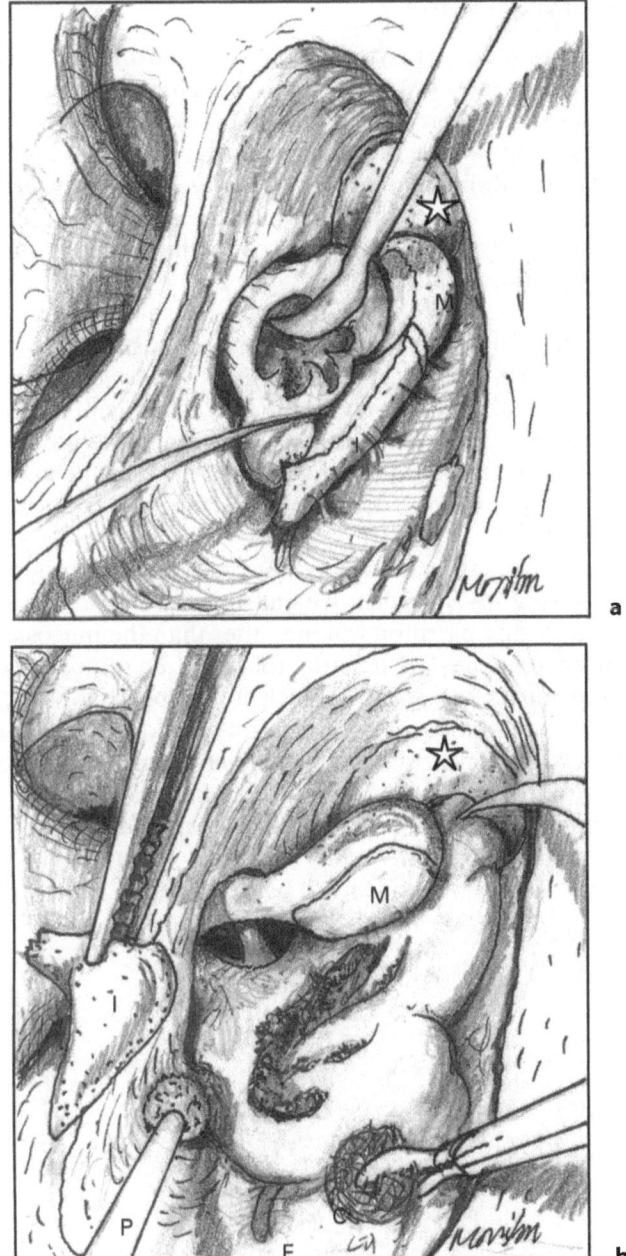

Fɪɢ. 3–3a,b. Eradication of cholesteatomatous matrix in (**a**) attic cholesteatoma and (**b**) adhesive cholesteatoma. *M*, malleus; *I*, incus; *C*, cotton ball; *P*, posterior tympanotomy; *F*, fistula of semicircular canal; *star*, anterior attic bony plate

3.2.5 Anterior Tympanotomy

Anterior tympanotomy starts in a search for the supratubal recess or the mucosal fold, to learn whether the bony partition is thick or thin (Fig. 3–4a). Then the anterior attic bony plate is removed with a diamond burr, beginning from its anterior inferior portion, where it is thinnest and even membranous in some cases (Fig. 3–4b). If the supratubal recess is large, a curved chisel specially designed for this operation is useful. The bony ledge must be removed completely, but the mucosa of the recess must be kept intact to cover the raw bony surface, if it is not found to be very pathological.

At the end of an anterior tympanotomy, the eustachian tube can be seen widely over the semicanal of the tensor tympani from the mastoid side (Fig. 3–5). If the recess is small and the bony partition is thick, removal of bony tissue during widening of the supratubal ventilation route may be difficult and may take a long time. This type of bony partition is called the pyramidal type; in such cases, the mucoperiosteum on the tubal side of the bony tissue must be kept intact (Fig. 3–6a) to be used later to cover raw bone to protect it from reclosure by formation of new bone (Fig. 3–6b).

In some cases, cholesteatoma develops anteriorly into the original space for the supratubal recess (Fig. 3–7a, right); we call this type the anterior type. In the anterior type, the closing partition is none other than the mucosal fold and bony plate of the tensor tympani. The mucosal fold must be removed (Fig. 3–7a, left), and the bony plate must be removed as much as possible (Fig. 3–7b, right and left). In all cases of cholesteatoma, special attention should be paid to the bony plate and mucosal fold of the tensor tympani, whether or not they close the supratubal ventilation route of the inferior border of the supratubal recess. If the bony plate is long and the mucosal fold is not perforated, they should be removed thoroughly, as shown in Fig. 3–7. I would classify the bony tissue removed by anterior tympanotomy into four types, which will be explained in Chapter 5.

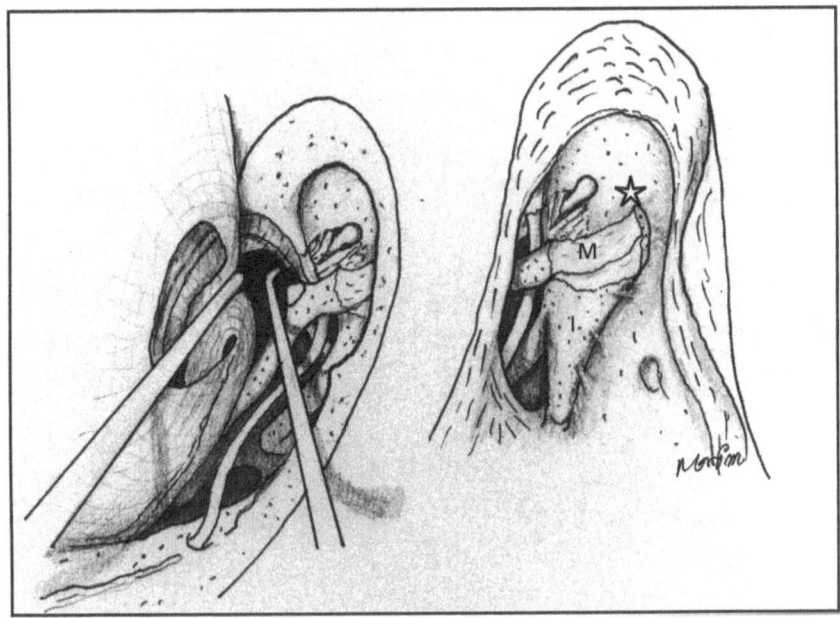

a

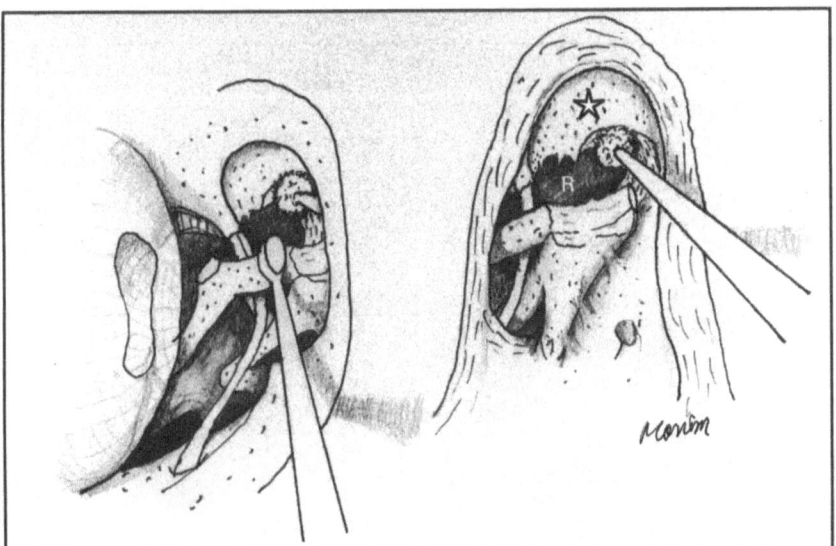

b

Fig. 3–4a,b. Beginning of anterior tympanotomy. **a** Exposure of the anterior attic bony plate and the anterior attic mucosal fold searched for, from tubal side. **b** Removal of the bony plate to open the supratubal recess. *left* (**a** and **b**) views from ear canal side, with left eye; *right* (**a** and **b**) views from mastoid side, with right eye. *R*, supratubal recess; *M*, malleus; *I*, incus; *star*, anterior attic bony plate

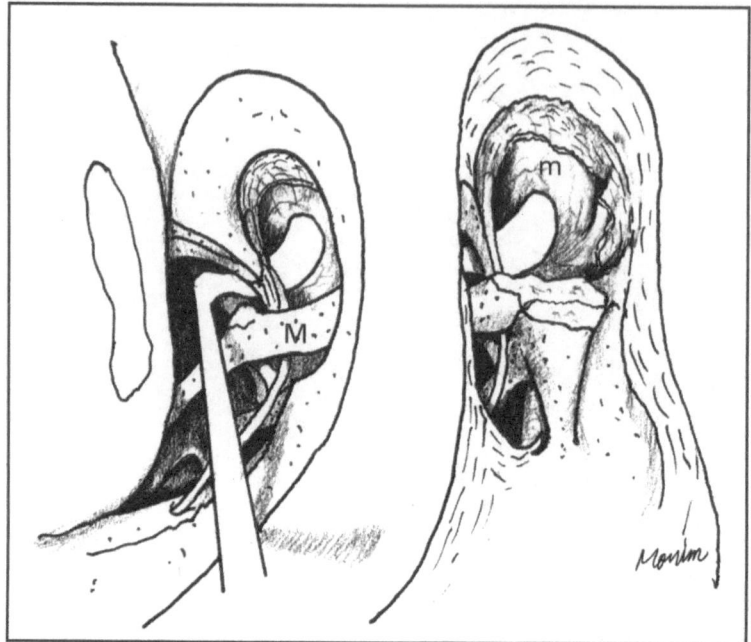

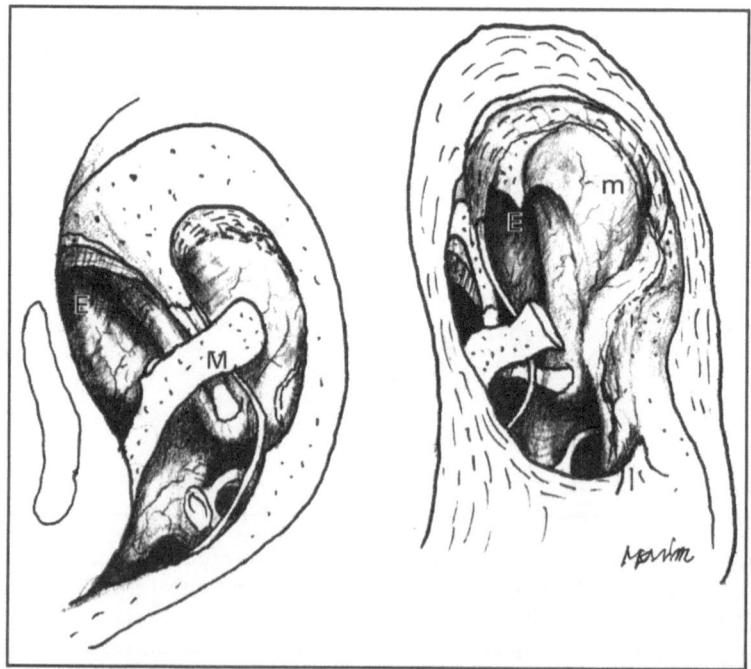

FɪG. 3–5a,b. Anterior tympanotomy of plate type. **a** Keeping the mucosa of the supratubal recess. **b** View at the end of anterior tympanotomy. *M*, malleus; *E*, eustachian tube; *m*, recess mucosa

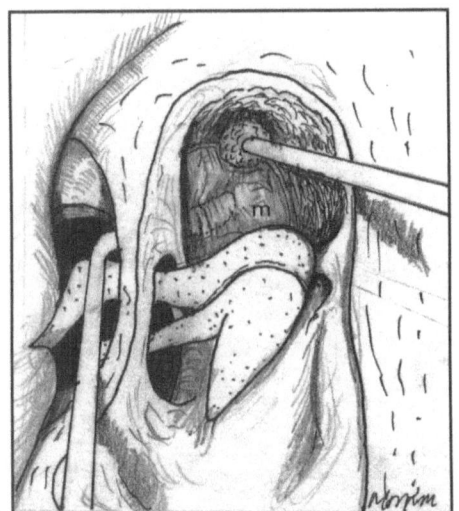
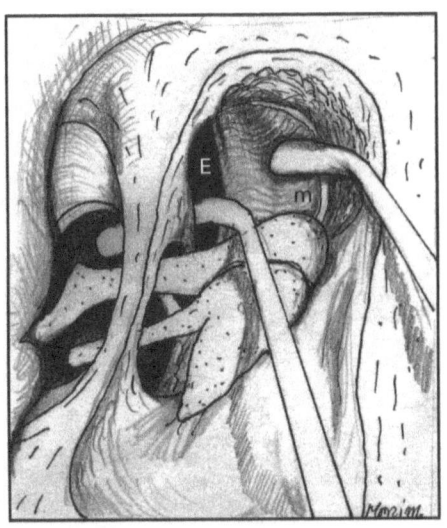

a   b

Fig. 3–6a,b. Anterior tympanotomy of pyramidal type. **a** Removal of massive bony tissue leaving the mucoperiosteum. **b** Covering raw bony surface with mucoperiosteum. *m*, mucoperiosteum; *E*, eustachian tube

3.2.6 Ossiculoplasty and Meatoplasty

Reconstruction of the ossicular chain is always done at the first surgery, and a second operation is not usually planned. For material we use autograft, as far as possible. The trimmed incudal body or short crus most frequently provide material for interposition between the malleus and the stapes or its footplate. The malleus must be kept intact, as far as possible; at least the malleal neck and handle with the tensor tendon must be kept in position in all cases, although a pathological malleal head may be removed.

Any large bony defect at the scutum is reconstructed using cortical bone chips covered by a free fascial graft from the temporal muscle. Any large defect of the posterior canal wall (spontaneous radical mastoidectomy) is reconstructed using bone chips covered by a split Palva's flap. In some cases of adhesive cholesteatoma, bare bony surfaces on the promontorium are covered with Gelfilm or Gelfoam, or with mucous membrane obtained from the mastoid antrum, if possible. We never insert a sheet of silicone. Defects in the eardrum are also closed with a free fascial graft. The retroauricular incision in the skin is sutured, usually without placement of any drain, but with use of a drain in cases with severe infection.

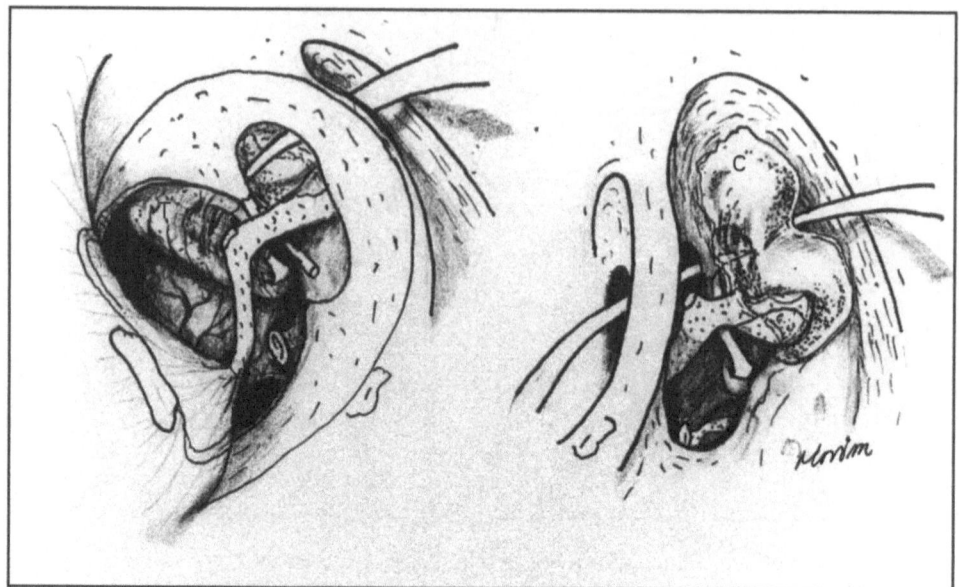

a

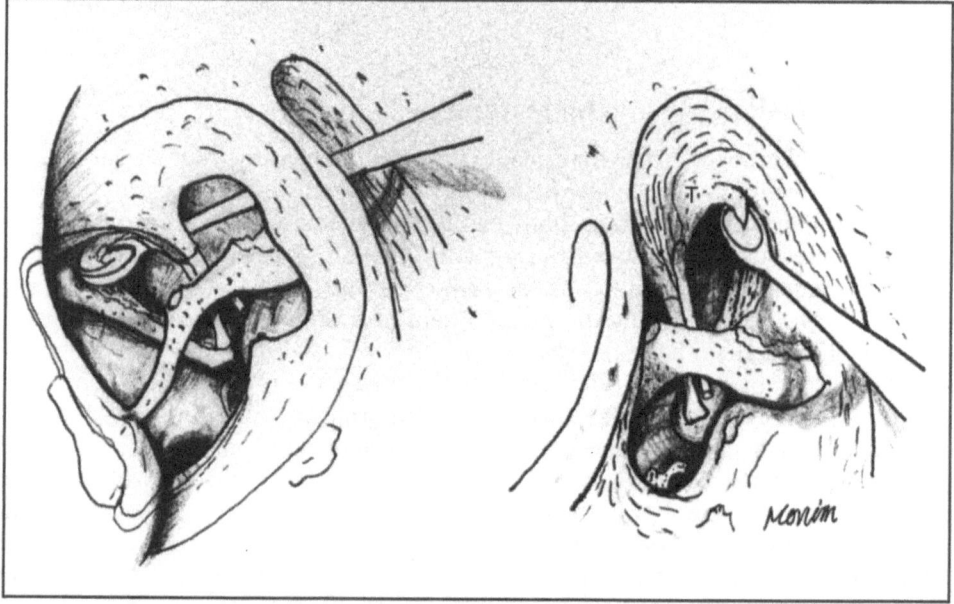

b

FIG. 3–7. Anterior tympanotomy of anterior type. **a** Removal of cholesteatomatous matrix in front of the malleus. **b** Removal of the tensor tympani bony plate. *C*, cholesteatomatous matrix; *T*, tensor tympani bony plate

3.2.7 Surgical Complications and Related Matters of Anterior Tympanotomy

A thorough knowledge of surgical anatomy around the supratubal recess is indispensable to avoiding surgical complications of anterior tympanotomy. Figure 3–8 illustrates the surgical anatomical view around the supratubal recess. The most important landmark is the facial nerve, which runs under the malleal head from the internal auditory meatus to the mastoid. If the bony wall of the labyrinth, under the malleal head, is not drilled there is no chance of damaging the facial nerve. In some cases the nerve may already be exposed when the bony wall has been absorbed by cholesteatoma. Exposure of the nerve itself during use of a diamond burr is not harmful. There is also a possibility that the greater petrosal nerve can be exposed at the tegmen tympani; we have, however, never seen such a case.

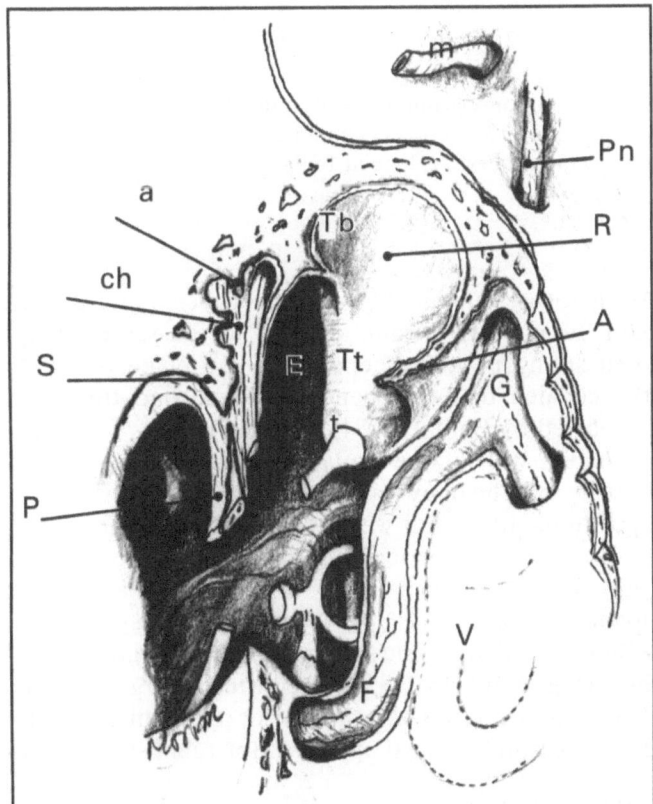

Fig. 3–8. Surgical anatomical view around the supratubal recess. *A*, anterior attic bony plate partially removed; *R*, supratubal recess; *E*, eustachian tube; *Tb*, tensor tympani bony plate; *Tt*, tensor tympani semicanal; *t*, tensor tympani tendon; *ch*, chorda tympani; *S*, anterior attic spine; *P*, anterior mallear process; *a*, anterior tympanic artery; *V*, lateral semicircular canal; *F*, facial nerve; *G*, geniculate ganglion; *m*, meningeal artery; *Pn*, superficial petrosal nerve

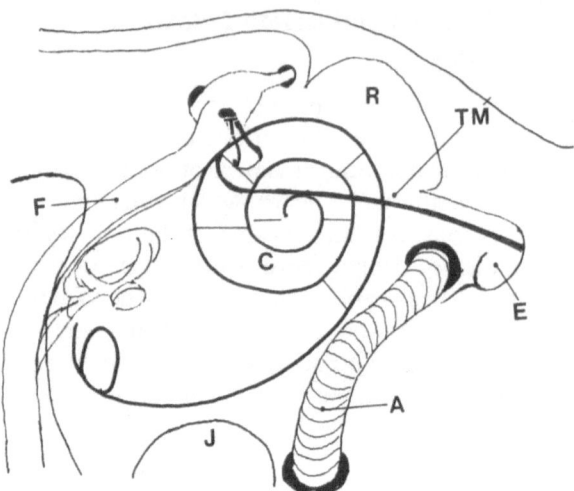

FIG. 3–9. Illustrative anatomy around the supratubal recess. *R*, supratubal recess; *C*, cochlea; *T*, tensor tendon; *TM*, tensor tympani semicanal; *A*, internal carotid artery; *E*, eustachian tube; *F*, facial nerve; *J*, jugular bulb

The cochlea is located under the supratubal recess and the semicanal of the tensor tympani. Its apex is 2–3 mm anterior to the tensor tympani tendon. If anterior tympanotomy is done deeper than the plane of the tensor tympani semicanal, the cochlea may be opened at its second turn, resulting in total deafness, as reported by Banfai (1984) (Fig. 3–9).

Under the medial wall of the protympanum near the tubal isthmus is the internal carotid artery. The bony wall covering the carotid is an average of 1.5 mm thick at this position, although it was found to be perforated in 2% of temporal bones studied by Savic and Dieric (1985). It is possible to open the semicanal of the tensor tympani, and the tensor tympani muscle may also be extracted during anterior tympanotomy, but this is not very harmful. The semicanal is an effective guide to reaching the tubal isthmus while avoiding damage to the carotid artery and the cochlea (Fig. 3–10). In 1985, we reported a surgical technique to open a closed tubal isthmus by removing the tensor tympani muscle; we called this procedure the musculotubal canal approach for tubal stenosis (Morimitsu et al. 1985).

In cases with extremely large cholesteatomas (Fig. 3–11), the facial nerve can be kept as a bony bridge without causing paresis. After pathological tissues have

--→

FIG. 3–11. Surgical view of extremely large cholesteatoma. *A*, widely exposed internal carotid artery; *T*, tensor tympani muscle; *F*, facial nerve kept in a bony bridge; *S*, sigmoid sinus; *I*, internal auditory meatus with the eighth cranial nerve

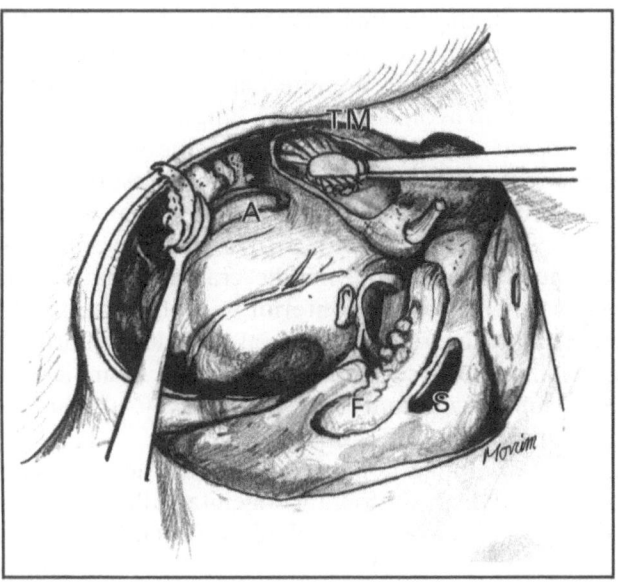

Fig. 3–10. Surgical view of the protympanum. *A*, internal carotid artery exposed by removal of pathological bone; *TM*, tensor tympani muscle exposed by opening the tensor tympani semicanal; *S*, fistula at the lateral semicircular canal; *F*, facial nerve exposed with pathological change

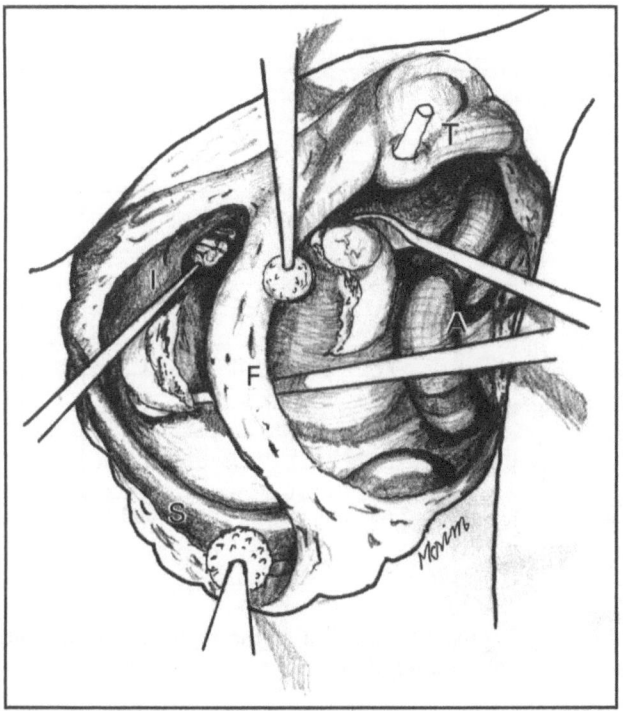

11

been totally eradicated, the internal carotid artery is exposed widely and the internal auditory meatus opened as the labyrinth is completely removed. It is important, in such cases, to plug the internal auditory meatus completely with bone wrapped in fascia to avoid long-lasting liquorrhea or intracranial infection.

The chorda tympani and the anterior tympanic artery run in the anterior mallear ligament and then in the tympanosquamous fissure, located at the lateral wall of the supratubal recess. They are often damaged during anterior tympanotomy, especially in cases with a pyramidal type of partitioned recess. Exposure of the dura mater of the middle cranial fossa may happen, causing leakage of cerebrospinal fluid at the anterior wall of the supratubal recess or the low tympanic tegmen. Closure with a fascial graft using fibrin glue is easy and useful. In conclusion, we have seen no cases of severe complication in surgery for cholesteatoma combined with anterior tympanotomy, although there are many important organs around the supratubal recess.

Concerning anterior tympanotomy itself, we experienced the interesting case of a 14-year-old girl in whom we found congenital adhesion of the malleal head and the anterior attic bony plate as described by Tos (1970). She visited our clinic, on November 27, 1990, because of speech retardation with nonprogressive bilat-

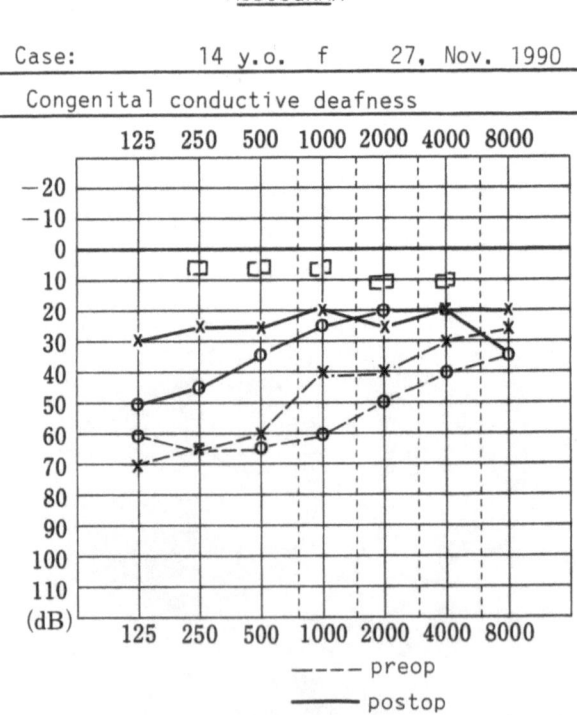

Fig. 3–12. Audiogram of congenital fixation of the malleus with an anterior attic bony plate, before and after surgical operation

eral hearing loss. Her pure-tone audiogram revealed bilateral severe conductive deafness with a stiff curve (Fig. 3–12). Tests of her aural reflexes revealed fixation of the ossicular chain with intact eardrums. Computerized tomographic examination (CT scan) of the temporal bone revealed bony conglutination of the malleus to the anterior attic bony plate bilaterally (Fig. 3–13).

The right ear was operated on using a transmeatal approach to atticotomy. The malleus was found completely fixed by bony adhesion to the anterior attic bony plate. This bony conglutination was released using chisels and curets to mobilize the ossicular chain. The left ear was operated on using anterior tympanotomy combined with an intact canal wall mastoidectomy. There was no inflammation and the tympanic isthmus was wide open (Fig. 3–14). After surgery, hearing was improved remarkably in the left ear and significantly in the right ear (see Fig. 3–12). These results indicate that anterior tympanotomy can be performed more completely by using a transmastoidal approach than by using a transmeatal approach.

This congenital malformation is very interesting because it represents remnants of the immature condition persisting after development of the mature individual. The malleus develops from Meckel's cartilage in mesenchymal tissue, in which the anterior attic bony plate also develops. In other words, the malleus and the bony plate arise from the same maternal tissue. It may be possible to say that they have a stage positioning very close together during development. Furthermore, we have described that the mucosal fold between the malleal head and the anterior attic bony plate is made by the bony plate changing into a mucosal fold during childhood; we called this the anterior attic mucosal fold. Findings in this surgical case seem to support our theory.

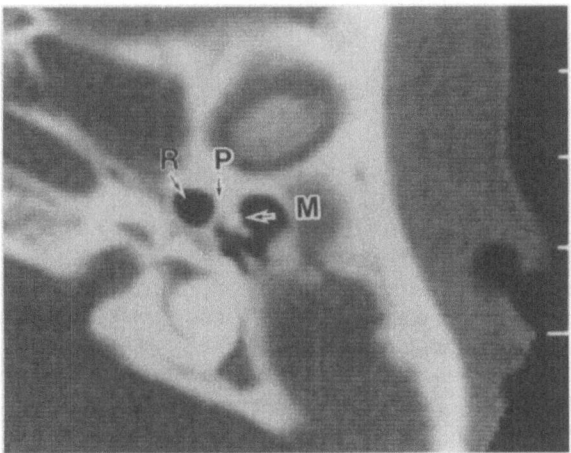

Fig. 3–13. Computed tomography (CT) scan of the temporal bone in congenital fixation of the malleus. *M*, malleus; *R*, supratubal recess; *P*, anterior attic bony plate

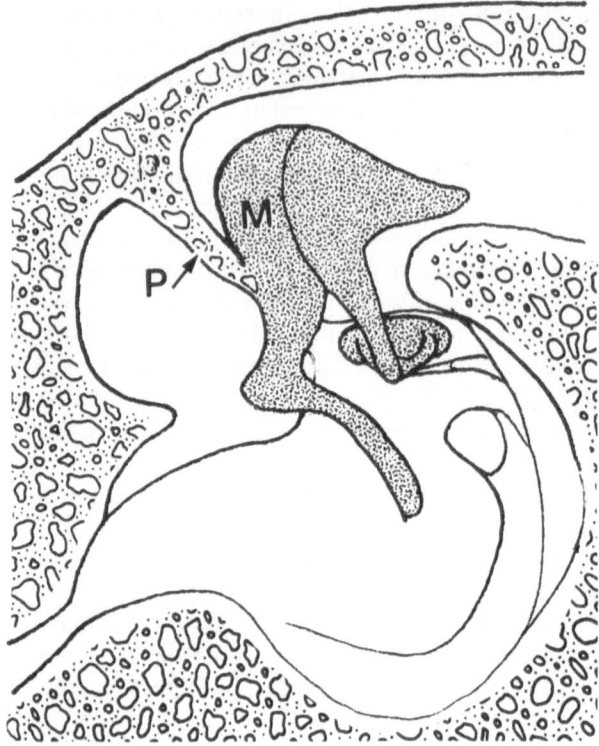

FIG. 3–14. Surgical findings in congenital fixation of the malleus with the anterior attic bony plate. *M*, mallear head; *P*, anterior attic bony plate

References

Banfai P (1984) Results with eight-channel cochlear implants. Adv Audiol 2:1–8

Bhide AR (1982) Combined approach tympanoplasty with lateral tympanotomy—a review of 42 cases. Auris Nasus Larynx (Tokyo) 9:1–7

Farrier JB (1982) The anterior attico-tympanotomy. Laryngoscope 76:768–779

Jansen C (1967) Posteriore Tympanotomie: Zugang zum Mittelohr mit Erhaltung des ausseren Gehoergangs. Arch Otolaryngol 188:2–6

Jansen C (1984) Cited in Deguine C (1984) Cholesteatoma surgery: what about the third intervention? In: Tos M, Thomsen J, Peiterson E (eds) Cholesteatoma and mastoid surgery. Kugler & Ghedini, Amsterdam, pp 821–825

Morimitsu T, Nagai T, Nagai M, Enatsu K, Ide M (1985) Musculotubal canal approach for stenotic eustachian tube. In: Marquet FE (ed) Surgery and pathology of the middle ear. Nijhoff, Boston, pp 52–56

Palva T (1973) Operative technique in mastoid obliteration. Acta Otolaryngol (Stockh) 75:289–290

Portmann M (1985) The choice of techniques of the surgery of chronic otitis media with cholesteatoma. J Laryngol Otol 89:533–547

Proctor B (1989) Surgical anatomy of the ear and temporal bone. Thieme, New York, pp 83–84

Sadé J (1982) Combined approach tympanoplasty in cholesteatoma surgery: a report on 1904 adults and 472 children. In: Sadé J (ed) Cholesteatoma and mastoid surgery. Kugler, Amsterdam, pp 491–493

Savic D, Dieric D (1985) Anatomical variations and relations in the medical wall of the bony portion of the eustachian tube. Acta Otolaryngol (Stockh) 99:551–556

Sheehy JL, Patterson ME (1967) Intact canal wall tympanoplasty with mastoidectomy. Laryngoscope 77:1502–1542

Smyth GD (1976) Postoperative cholesteatoma in combined approach tympanoplasty. J Laryngol Otol 90:597–621

Suzuki J (1982) Tympanoplasty from type I to type 0 (in Japanese). Igaku-Shoin Tokyo

Tos M (1970) Bony fixation of the malleus and incus. Acta Otolaryngol (Stockh) 70:95–104

Tos M (1982) Modification of combined approach tympanoplasty in attic cholesteatoma. Arch Otolaryngol Head Neck Surg 108:772–778

Wullstein SR (1974) Osteoplastic epitympanotomy. Ann Otol Rhinol Laryngol 83:663–668

Zini C, Bacciu S, Sandellari R, Pasanisi E (1989) Intra-operative management of the osseous eustachian tube: techniques and results. In: Tos M, Thomsen J, Peiterson E (eds) Cholesteatoma and mastoid surgery. Kugler & Ghedini, Amsterdam, pp 533–541

Chapter 4
Clinical Results of Anterior Tympanotomy in Surgery for Cholesteatoma

4.1 Recurrent and Residual Cholesteatoma

Diagnostic criteria for *recurrent* cholesteatoma are as follows: (1) the patient will have undergone a previous surgical procedure to treat attic or adhesive cholesteatoma; (2) the same type of cholesteatoma is then found during reoperation; (3) the cholesteatoma clearly communicates with the retracted pars flaccida or pars tensa.

Criteria for *residual* cholesteatoma are as follows: (1) the patient will have undergone a previous surgical procedure to treat attic or adhesive cholesteatoma; (2) cholesteatoma is then found in the middle-ear space at reoperation, but this has no direct communication with the new eardrum.

Anterior tympanotomy is not meant as a surgical procedure for eradication of pathological tissues that may evolve to residual cholesteatoma, but rather for improvement of intratympanic ventilation to prevent recurrent cholesteatoma. So, here we mainly analyze and discuss surgical results concerning recurrence. Eight surgeons operated on the patients studied for this purpose. They had experience in surgery for cholesteatoma that varied from 3 to 10 years and averaged 8 years, except for Dr. Morimitsu, who has more than 25 years of experience in this kind of procedure.

4.1.1 Attic Cholesteatoma Operated on Without Anterior Tympanotomy

Among 72 cases of attic cholesteatoma for which patients underwent operations during the 5 years between 1977 and 1982, 52 were analyzed. The surgical techniques used were canal-up, canal-down with reconstruction, and canal-down (only) methods. Selection of the method to be used was left to each surgeon according to intraoperative findings, although for small lesions without severe infection they tended to choose the canal-up method. Reconstruction of the posterior canal wall was done using autograft or homograft bone chips or cartilage. Postoperative follow-up time of primarily operated cases varied from 8 to 13

TABLE 4–1. Surgical results in cases of primary attic cholesteatoma without anterior tympanotomy

Method	Recurrence	Residual disease
Canal-up (67.2%)	10/37 (27.6%)	2/37 (5.4%)
Reconstruction (9.6%)	1/5 (20.0%)	1/5 (20.0%)
Canal-down (19.2%)	1/10 (10.0%)	1/10 (10.0%)
Totals	12/52 (23.0%)	4/52 (7.7%)

TABLE 4–2. Surgical results in reoperated cases of attic cholesteatoma without anterior tympanotomy

Method	Recurrence	Residual disease
Canal-up	3/5 (60.0%)	3/4 (75.5%)
Reconstruction	0/1 (0%)	
Canal-down	0/3 (0%)	1/1 (100.0%)
Totals	3/9 (30.0%)	4/5 (80.0%)

years. Recurrent or residual cholesteatoma was confirmed by reoperation. The results in primary and reoperated cases are shown in Tables 4–1 and 4–2.

The canal-up method was used in 67.2% of all cases, and the rate of recurrence for these patients was 27.6%. Rates of recurrence in the group with reconstructions and the group undergoing canal-down procedures were 20.0% and 10.0%, respectively. Overall, recurrent cholesteatoma occurred in 23.0% and residual cholesteatoma in 7.7%.

Rates of recurrence in patients undergoing canal-up procedures and reconstructions were higher than rates in the group undergoing canal-down procedures. Recurrences occurred in 27.6% of the group who had undergone canal-up procedures for primary lesions and in 60% of the reoperated recurrence group. This means that the canal-up procedure used at that time does not offer proper protection against recurrence and reoperation. In other words, this technique did not remove the cause of retraction and subsequent recurrent cholesteatoma.

Cases of residual cholesteatoma after reoperation were all in children. It is therefore possible to say that complete removal of pathological tissues remaining at reoperation was very difficult to attain in children by using the canal-up method. Three recurrent and four residual cases were operated on for a third time, using the reconstructive method, with acceptable results.

4.1.2 Attic Cholesteatoma Operated on with Anterior Tympanotomy

During the period from 1982 to 1994, all 163 of our cases of attic cholesteatoma were operated on consistently using the canal-up method combined with anterior tympanotomy, without considerations of size of cholesteatoma, presence of inflammation or tubal dysfuncion, or age of the patient. Recurrent cases that had been operated on in other hospitals using the canal-up technique but without anterior tympanotomy were also included here as primary cases, because this was the first use of anterior tympanotomy; this applied to 27 of the 163 cases (16.5%). We also analyzed 20 cases of recurrent cholesteatoma that had been operated on in other hospitals using the canal-up method with anterior tympanotomy.

The drilled mastoid cavity was not obliterated but kept as a cavity. Large defects of the scutum were closed using bone chips or auricular cartilage and fibrin glue. No silicone sheets were used in the tympanic cavity. The retroauricular incision was sutured primarily without placement of any drain, except in a few cases that had severe inflammation. Results concerning recurrent and residual cholesteatoma in primary and reoperated cases are shown in Tables 4–3 and 4–4, respectively. The distribution by age of attic retraction without debris, recurrence, or residue is shown in Table 4–5.

The rate of recurrence was decreased significantly, from 27.0% to 9.8% in primary cases and from 60% to 16.7% in reoperated cases, by using anterior tympanotomy combined with the canal-up method. The period until reoperation ranged from 15 to 90 months, with an average of 64 months in cases that had received the combined surgery originally. Patients in the group who had

TABLE 4–3. Surgical results in primary operations for attic cholesteatoma with anterior tympanotomy

Method	Recurrence	Residual disease
Canal-up	16/163 (9.8%)	12/163 (7.4%)

TABLE 4–4. Surgical results in recurrent cases of attic cholesteatoma with anterior tympanotomy

Method	Recurrence	Residual disease
Canal-up	6/36 (16.7%)	3/36 (8.3%)

Results include 20 cases operated on in other hospitals.

TABLE 4–5. Distribution by age of patient with attic retraction, recurrence, and residual disease after anterior tympanotomy

Age (yr)	~9	10–19	20–29	30–39	40–49	50–59	60+	Total
Number of cases	21	31	11	22	38	27	13	163
Retraction	3	5	1	2	5	1	1	18
Recurrence	3	5	1	4	1	2	0	16
Residual disease	2	6	0	0	1	3	0	12

undergone canal-up procedures without anterior tympanotomy had all been selected because their small cholesteatomas had no active inflammation. Therefore, results obtained for the group who had received anterior tympanotomy initially must be evaluated more closely because these ears had been in worse condition than those in the group who had not received anterior tympanotomy initially.

Retraction of the attic without debris was observed in 11.0% of our 163 cases. Distribution of retractions and recurrences were very similar in all age groups. Cases with retractions must be followed carefully, even though their retraction may be stable and demonstrate self-cleansing function and a visible bottom.

The 16 recurrent cases were examined more precisely. Recurrences occurred in 15.3% of patients younger than 19 years old, although the rate in patients more than 20 years old fell to 7.2%. Six of the 16 recurrent cases (37.5%) were in ears that had been operated on before in other hospitals without use of anterior tympanotomy. Eleven of the 16 cases (68.5%) had been operated on originally by surgeons with less experience. Three cases in children under 9 years of age had copious discharge caused by severe inflammation, tubal dysfunction with glue, and membranous closure of the supratubal route by a remnant of the tensor tympani mucosal fold or by scar tissue, confirmed at reoperation. In a child of 3 years, the posterior canal wall had to be taken down because of recurrence caused by severe inflammation after reoperation. This was the only case in which the posterior ear canal was surgically removed. Thus the final rate for preservation of the external ear canal intact was 99.4% in cases of attic cholesteatoma.

In eight adult cases, the cause of recurrence was (1) incomplete removal of a pyramidal type of bony partition or occlusion of the supratubal route by formation of new bone of (in four cases) a tympanosclerotic mass; (2) inadequate surgical procedure that had left the tensor tympani fold in three cases; and (3) bony closure of the eustachian tube, which failed to keep the lumen open, in one case. These kinds of problems should be preventable through technical advancement of surgeons. In fact, the rates of clinical recurrence significantly decreased from 18% during the period from 1983 to 1991 to 3% during the period from 1991 to 1993, indicating improvement in surgical technique in using anterior tympanotomy.

The rate of rerecurrence in attic cholesteatoma was 16.7%. These six cases were all third operations using the same method. Two cases showed retraction after reoperation because of poor tubal function, so tubes in the eardrum were inevitable. The other four cases were in acceptable condition. The rate of residual attic cholesteatoma after primary procedures without anterior tympanotomy was 7.7%; in groups who underwent anterior tympanotomy, residual disease occurred in 7.4% after the primary procedure and in 8.3% after reoperation, a rate that is roughly equal because anterior tympanotomy is not a surgical procedure for the eradication of pathological tissue.

TABLE 4–6. Surgical results in cases of primary adhesive cholesteatoma without anterior tympanotomy

Method	Recurrence	Residual disease
Canal-up (66.7%)	5/18 (27.8%)	1/18 (5.6%)
Reconstruction (11.1%)	2/3 (66.7%)	0/3 (0%)
Canal-down (22.2%)	1/6 (16.7%)	2/6 (33.3%)
Totals	8/27 (29.6%)	3/27 (11.1%)

TABLE 4–7. Surgical results in reoperated cases of adhesive cholesteatoma without anterior tympanotomy

Method	Recurrence	Residual disease
Canal-up	2/6 (33.3%)	2/6 (33.3%)
Reconstruction	1/1 (100%)	0/1 (0%)
Canal-down	0/1 (0%)	0/1 (0%)
Totals	3/8 (37.5%)	2/8 (25.0%)

4.1.3 Adhesive Cholesteatoma Operated on Without Anterior Tympanotomy

Among our 32 cases of adhesive cholesteatoma operated on without anterior tympanotomy during the period from 1977 to 1982, 27 cases were analyzed. The method selected, surgical techniques used, and average follow-up time were the same as those for patients with attic cholesteatoma. Results are shown in Tables 4–6 and 4–7. The canal-up method was used in 18 of 27 cases (66.7%), and the rate of recurrence in these patients was 27.8%. Rates of recurrence in patients undergoing reconstructive and canal-down procedures were 66.7% and 16.7%, respectively. The overall rate of recurrence was 29.6%, and residual cholesteatoma was found in 11.1%. The external ear canal was preserved in 21 of 27 (77.8%). Results in the reoperated group were disappointing using either the canal-up or the reconstructive methods, although it was impossible to draw final conclusions because the number of cases was too small.

4.1.4 Adhesive Cholesteatoma Operated on with Anterior Tympanotomy

During the period from 1982 to 1994, 61 cases of adhesive cholesteatoma were operated on using the canal-up method combined with anterior tympanotomy. No cases had been operated on previously in other hospitals without using

TABLE **4–8.** Surgical results in primary operations for adhesive cholesteatoma with anterior tympanotomy

Method	Recurrence	Residual disease
Canal-up	5/61 (8.2%)	4/61 (6.5%)

TABLE **4–9.** Surgical results in reoperated cases of adhesive cholesteatoma with anterior tympanotomy

Method	Recurrence	Residual disease
Canal-up	1/7 (14.2%)	1/3 (33.3%)
Reconstruction	0/1 (0%)	0/1 (0%)
Total	1/8 (12.5%)	1/4 (25.0%)

Results include three cases operated on in other hospitals.

TABLE **4–10.** Distribution by age of patients with attic retraction, recurrence, and residual disease after anterior tympanotomy

Age (yr)	~9	10–19	20–29	30–39	40–49	50–59	60+	Total
Number of cases	7	8	2	8	17	15	4	61
Retraction	0	0	0	1	0	1	0	2
Recurrence	1	1	0	1	1	0	1	5
Residual disease	1	2	0	0	1	0	0	4

anterior tympanotomy, but 3 cases had been operated on in other hospitals using anterior tympanotomy; these were included in our reoperated cases. Results concerning recurrent and residual cholesteatoma after primary and reoperative procedures are shown in Tables 4–8 and 4–9.

Distributions by age of retractions in the posterior superior quadrant without debris, recurrence, or residue are shown in Table 4–10. The rate of recurrence was decreased significantly by using the combination procedure with anterior tympanotomy, from 27.8% to 8.2% in primary procedures and from 42.8% to 12.5% in reoperations. Retraction of the adhered eardrum without debris was observed in two cases (3.3%) in patients in their thirties and fifties. These cases must be followed up carefully. There were no special distributions by age reflected in recurrent and residual cholesteatoma.

Recurrent cases were examined more precisely. Recurrence of adhesive cholesteatoma occurred with no special distribution by age. Four of the five cases had been operated on by surgeons with less experience. Causes of recurrence included the following: (1) inadequate anterior tympanotomy that left the tensor tympani fold, in three cases; (2) incomplete removal of bony tissue in the anterior attic in one case; and (3) tubal dysfunction with glue, in two children. The rates of residual disease in those with and those without anterior tympanotomy were 6.5% and 11.1%, respectively, with no significant differences. One case rerecurred because of poor tubal function, even though adenoidectomy and tonsillectomy had been performed; this patient continues to be monitored.

4.1.5 Discussion

Recurrence of cholesteatoma is the most important problem in surgery for cholesteatoma that uses the canal-up method. Recurrence is simply caused by continuation of the pathogenic factors in cholesteatoma after the first operation. Although there is no agreed theory on the pathogenesis of acquired cholesteatoma, we believe that the real pathogenesis occurs in the region removed by anterior tympanotomy, because our rate of recurrence has been decreased significantly by using a combined procedure that incorporates anterior tympanotomy. For precise analysis of recurrent cases, it is first necessary to perform complete anterior tympanotomies.

Procedures on pyramidal types of partitions must be surgically complete so that the supratubal ventilation route is made as large as possible. Young surgeons especially must persevere in efforts to remove bony tissue completely as far as possible. In some recurrent cases, the tensor tympani partition had been left but the anterior attic partition removed completely. Children with severe infections or tubal dysfunction are not good candidates for the canal-up method, even when it is combined with anterior tympanotomy, especially not in cases with attic cholesteatoma. They must first be treated conservatively and then operated on using the canal-up method, but with planning for a second operation.

The canal-down method should not be used in children because a child's temporal bone is still developing, and use of a canal-down operation would frequently result in a troublesome mastoid later. Residual cholesteatoma that is caused by incomplete eradication of the matrix membrane has no direct relationship with anterior tympanochtomy that we have observed in our clinical results. Of course, removal of cholesteatoma matrix is more difficult when using canal-up methods than when using canal-down methods.

Strategies in surgery for cholesteatoma must aim at complete eradication of cholesteatomatous tissue and at improvement of intratympanic ventilation through the tympanic diaphragm using anterior tympanotomy. If eradication is not complete, then residual cholesteatoma will be inevitable even after anterior tympanotomy. If, on the other hand, ventilation is not completely achieved, cholesteatoma will inevitably recur, even after complete removal of pathological tissue. For cholesteatoma to be finally cured, both procedures must be done completely.

4.2 Comparative Postoperative Effects on Hearing After Anterior Tympanotomy or After Other Surgical Procedures for Cholesteatoma

The aims of surgery for cholesteatoma are (1) no recurrence of cholesteatoma, (2) no residual cholesteatoma, (3) a normal external ear canal with self-cleansing function, and (4) restoration of hearing to the level socially indicated, if possible. As a surgical procedure, anterior tympanotomy aims to fulfill (1) and (3), not to improve hearing. Its effects on hearing, however, especially when combined with an intact canal wall mastoidectomy, were studied. We used pure-tone audiograms from 91 ears that had attic and adhesive cholesteatoma operated on during the 7 years between 1987 and 1993. All cases had a favorable postoperative course without any recurrent or residual cholesteatoma and had not had subsequent ossiculoplasty to improve hearing.

Pure-tone audiograms taken directly before and about 1 year after the surgery were reviewed. Mean levels for air-conducted hearing at seven frequencies (125, 250, 500, 1000, 2000, 4000, and 8000 Hz); mean levels for air- and bone-conducted hearing in speech frequencies (500, 1000, and 2000 Hz), and pre- and postoperative levels for air- and bone-conducted hearing at 4000 Hz were calculated and compared statistically.

4.2.1 Levels of Air-Conducted Hearing in Attic Cholesteatoma

Types of ossiculoplasty performed were classified for 71 ears with attic cholesteatoma: 26 ears had undergone type I ossiculoplasty, 32 ears type III (including interposition between the malleus and the stapedial head), and 13 ears type IV (including interposition between the malleus and the stapedial footplate). In Table 4–11, mean pre- and postoperative levels for air-conducted hearing (with standard deviations), and the increments between pre- and postoperative levels (with standard deviations) are shown for each of seven frequencies in three types of ossiculoplasty.

4.2.1.1 Type I Ossiculoplasty

In this group, postoperative hearing levels were better by 5.8–8.8 dB than preoperative hearing levels at all seven frequencies (shown in column labeled "Increment"). The increments showed small improvements in middle frequencies; they were best at 1000 Hz, poorest at 125 Hz, and second-best at 4000 Hz. The mean preoperative hearing level at the seven frequencies was 37.5 dB ($\pm$14.2 dB), and the mean postoperative hearing level was 29.0 dB ($\pm$13.9 dB). The difference between these means was 8.4 dB ($\pm$13.9 dB) and was statistically significant at $P < .01$. Among 26 ears, postoperative hearing became worse in 2. As their levels for bone-conducted hearing were maintained at the same level after surgery, disruption of the ossicular chain was considered as a possible cause for the poorer air-conducted levels.

TABLE 4-11. Pre- and postoperative mean hearing levels (with SD) at seven frequencies, and the increments between them (with SD), in attic cholesteatoma

Frequency (Hz)	Preoperative X̄ (dB)	SD	Postoperative X̄ (dB)	SD	Increment X̄ (dB)	SD
Results in group who received type I ossiculoplasty ($n = 26$)						
125	39.6	12.2	33.9	17.1	5.8	15.7
250	40.2	14.4	33.1	15.2	7.1	13.8
500	38.5	14.3	30.8	13.5	7.7	12.8
1000	39.0	15.5	30.2	15.2	8.8	15.2
2000	33.3	14.4	25.0	14.3	8.3	12.6
4000	36.9	16.7	31.0	18.3	6.0	13.3
8000	50.4	25.7	42.1	22.5	8.3	14.7
Results in group who received type III ossiculoplasty ($n = 32$)						
125	53.9	12.8	46.4	17.1	7.5	15.1
250	55.2	15.7	46.3	18.2	8.9	18.0
500	52.8	15.2	43.6	18.8	9.2	20.6
1000	49.1	14.5	40.3	17.5	8.8	16.5
2000	46.4	15.2	36.1	20.0	10.3	17.0
4000	50.5	14.2	44.2	22.6	6.3	20.7
8000	58.8	22.3	59.1	26.3	−0.3	19.2
Results in group who received type IV ossiculoplasty ($n = 13$)						
125	64.6	12.0	57.3	12.5	7.3	13.8
250	65.0	13.5	56.9	14.9	8.1	14.4
500	60.0	14.7	53.5	13.6	6.5	13.6
1000	59.6	17.5	50.8	16.8	8.8	16.1
2000	48.5	15.9	40.8	18.8	7.7	12.4
4000	52.7	17.3	48.5	17.8	4.2	9.3
8000	58.9	23.1	50.0	18.3	8.8	10.8

4.2.1.2 Type III Ossiculoplasty

In this group, postoperative hearing levels were better by 6.3–10.3 dB over preoperative hearing levels, except at 8000 Hz. The increments were best at 2000 Hz and poorest at 8000 Hz; second-best fell at 4000 Hz. Mean preoperative hearing levels at seven frequencies were 49.3 dB (±13.4 dB), and mean postoperative hearing levels were 40.1 dB (±17.0 dB). The difference between those two means was 9.3 dB (±16.2 dB), statistically significant at $P < .01$. Among 32 ears, 2 showed increase in the air–bone gap because of failure in ossiculoplasty, and one (with mixed deafness) showed aggravation of the bone-conducted hearing loss because of damage to the inner ear during surgery.

4.2.1.3 Type IV Ossiculoplasty

In this group, postoperative hearing levels were 4.2–8.8 dB better than preoperative hearing levels at all seven frequencies. The increments were best at 1000 Hz and 8000 Hz and poorest at 4000 Hz. Mean preoperative hearing levels at the seven frequencies were 56.9 dB (±14.9 dB), and mean postoperative levels were 48.9 dB (±15.1 dB). The difference between these means was 8.0 dB (±13.1 dB), statistically significant at $P < .05$. Among 13 ears, only 1 showed decreased bone-conducted hearing function.

4.2.2 Levels of Air-Conducted Hearing in Adhesive Cholesteatoma

Similar studies were done on 20 ears with adhesive cholesteatoma: 4 with type I, 11 with type III, and 5 with type IV ossiculoplasty (Table 4–12 and in Figs. 4–1 and 4–2).

4.2.2.1 Type I Ossiculoplasty

In this group, postoperative hearing levels were from 3.8 to 16.3 dB better than

TABLE 4–12. Pre- and postoperative mean hearing levels (with SD) at seven frequencies, and the increments between them (with SD), in adhesive cholesteatoma

Frequency (Hz)	Preoperative X̄ (dB)	SD	Postoperative X̄ (dB)	SD	Increment X̄ (dB)	SD
Results in group who received type I ossiculoplasty ($n = 4$)						
125	45.0	17.8	31.3	13.2	13.8	10.3
250	46.3	19.7	30.0	10.8	16.3	9.5
500	35.0	20.4	27.5	6.5	7.5	15.6
1000	31.3	17.0	25.0	8.2	6.3	17.0
2000	30.0	15.8	16.3	4.8	13.8	13.8
4000	28.8	20.6	18.8	6.3	10.0	15.8
8000	35.0	12.3	31.3	6.3	3.8	9.5
Results in group who received type III ossiculoplasty ($n = 11$)						
125	57.7	20.3	48.6	19.9	9.1	17.4
250	62.7	22.5	48.2	26.6	14.6	15.7
500	56.8	23.3	51.8	30.1	5.0	17.3
1000	51.4	19.0	52.7	29.2	−1.4	21.7
2000	46.8	22.7	45.9	28.5	0.9	18.0
4000	53.6	26.8	49.1	25.2	4.5	14.6
8000	60.0	27.4	56.8	29.3	3.2	15.4
Results in group who received type IV ossiculoplasty ($n = 5$)						
125	61.0	10.8	67.0	11.5	−6.0	8.2
250	61.0	14.3	69.0	19.5	−8.0	22.5
500	56.0	13.9	62.0	14.4	−6.0	15.6
1000	48.0	11.5	52.0	14.8	−4.0	6.5
2000	50.0	10.6	48.0	18.6	2.0	14.0
4000	60.0	11.2	61.0	19.2	−1.0	20.4
8000	81.0	8.9	79.0	23.0	2.0	15.3

FIG. 4–1a–c. Preoperative (*squares*) and postoperative (*circles*) mean hearing level (with SD) at seven frequencies, and the increments between them (with SD), in attic cholesteatoma. **a** Results in group who received type I ossiculoplasty. **b** Results in group who received type III ossiculoplasty. **c** Results in group who received type IV ossiculoplasty

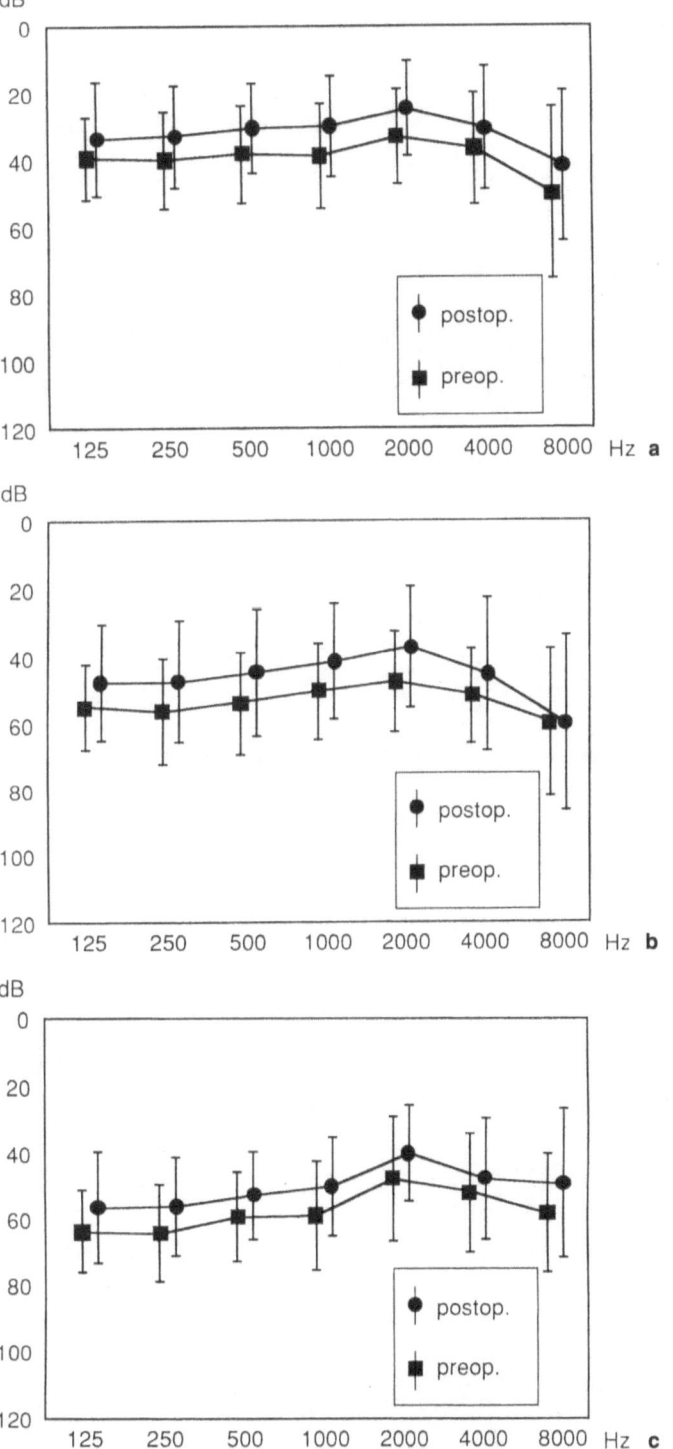

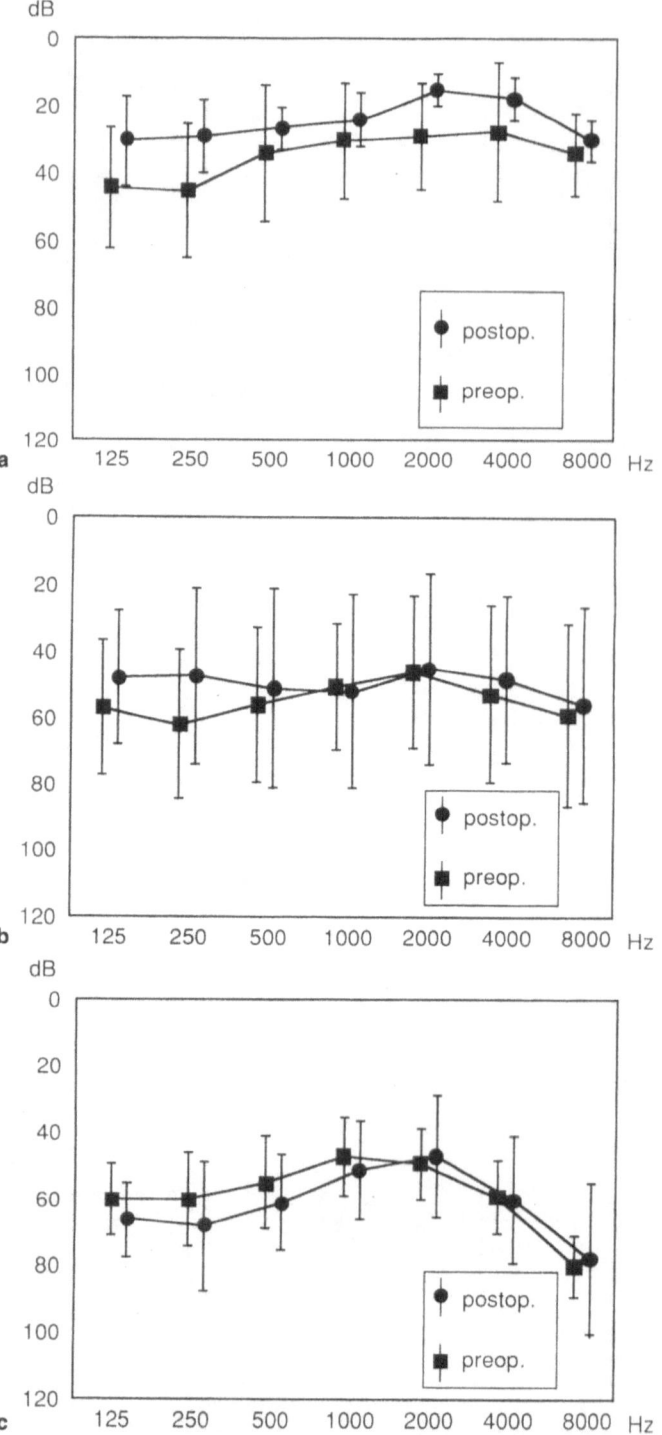

preoperative hearing levels for all seven frequencies. The best increment was 16.3 dB at 250 Hz and the poorest 3.8 dB at 8000 Hz. Mean preoperative hearing levels at the seven frequencies were 31.9 dB (±17.4 dB), and mean postoperative hearing levels were 23.4 dB (±6.4 dB). The difference between these means was 8.4 dB (±15.6 dB), but this was not statistically significant. No cases showed decrease in postoperative hearing.

4.2.2.2 Type III Ossiculoplasty

In this group, the differences from preoperative to postoperative hearing levels at seven frequencies were distributed between a loss of 1.4 dB and a gain of 14.6 dB. The best increment was 14.6 dB at 250 Hz, the worst a loss of 1.4 dB at 1000 Hz. Mean preoperative hearing levels for the seven frequencies were 51.6 dB (±19.7 dB), and mean postoperative levels were 50.8 dB (±28.7 dB). The difference between these means was 0.8 dB (±19.0 dB), which was not statistically significant. Among these 11 ears, 8 had high or moderate degrees of mixed deafness before surgery, and 2 of these showed aggravation of a bone-conducted hearing loss after surgery.

4.2.2.3 Type IV Ossiculoplasty

In this group, the differences from preoperative to postoperative hearing levels were distributed from a loss of 8.0 dB to a gain of 2.0 dB at the seven frequencies. The best increment was 2.0 dB at 2000 Hz and 8000 Hz, and the worst loss was 8.0 dB at 250 Hz. Mean preoperative hearing levels at the seven frequencies were 50.5 dB (±11.4 dB), and mean postoperative levels were 53.5 dB (±13.6 dB). Postoperative hearing decreased in all cases in this group, although the differences of −3.0 dB (±7.5 dB) were not statistically significant.

Among these five ears, three had a high degree of mixed deafness preoperatively, and one showed aggravation of a bone-conducted hearing loss at 250 and at 500 Hz after surgery.

4.2.3 Levels of Air- and Bone-Conducted Hearing as These Relate to Speech Frequencies

From the mean pre- and postoperative levels of air- and bone-conducted hearing at speech frequencies (500, 1000, and 2000 Hz), we calculated increments in hearing for each type of ossiculoplasty (Fig. 4–3). Increments are shown in numerals beside each square or triangle sign at the middle of the bars.

←——————————————————————————————

Fɪɢ. 4–2a–c. Preoperative (*squares*) and postoperative (*circles*) mean hearing levels (with SD) at seven frequencies, and the increments between them (with SD), in adhesive cholesteatoma. **a** Results in group who received type I ossiculoplasty. **b** Results in group who received type III ossiculoplasty. **c** Results in group who received type IV ossiculoplasty

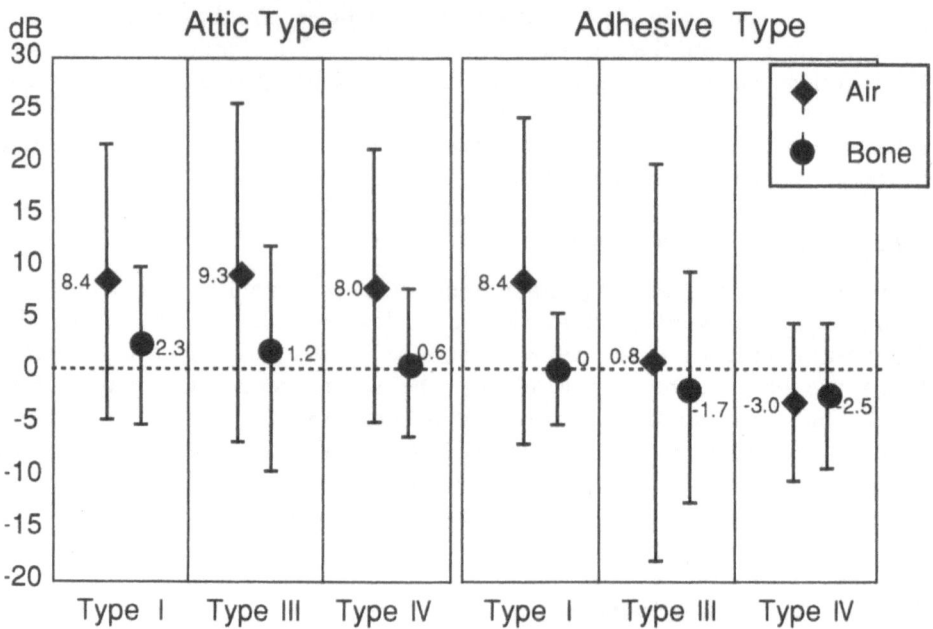

Fig. 4-3. Gains in air- (*diamonds*) and bone-conductive (*circles*) hearing at speech frequencies in each type of ossiculoplasty for attic (*left*) and adhesive (*right*) cholesteatoma

4.2.3.1 Attic Cholesteatoma

In attic cholesteatoma, gains in air-conducted hearing after surgery (for each type of ossiculoplasty) were 8.4, 9.3, and 8.0 dB, respectively; gains in bone-conducted hearing were 2.3, 1.2, and 0.6 dB, respectively. There were no clear differences between frequencies. Large increments in air-conducted hearing and small increments in bone-conducted hearing in the group with attic cholesteatoma meant that the air–bone gap had clearly decreased. On the other hand, small increments in both air- and bone-conducted hearing in groups with adhesive cholesteatoma undergoing types III and IV ossiculoplasty meant that no decrease in the air–bone gap was achieved by surgery. The most interesting result was improvement in the bone-conducted hearing level after surgery, although these values were not very high. In all, 63.4% of 71 ears showed an air–bone gap within 20 dB postoperatively.

4.2.3.2 Adhesive Cholesteatoma

In adhesive cholesteatoma, gains in air-conducted hearing were 8.4 dB for type I and 0.8 dB for type III ossiculoplasty, but there was a loss of 3.0 dB with type IV ossiculoplasty. Concerning bone-conducted hearing, there was no gain with type

I and losses of 1.7 dB with type III and 2.5 dB with type IV. Although none of these changes was statistically significant, levels of bone-conducted hearing for all in the groups receiving types III and IV ossiculoplasty became worse. In all, 45% of 20 ears with adhesive cholesteatoma showed an air–bone gap within 20 dB post-operatively.

4.2.4 Bone-Conducted Hearing at 4000 Hz

During anterior tympanotomy, surgery is also performed near the supratubal recess in front of the malleal head, using burrs or chisels. There is a danger, therefore, of damage to the inner ear from the burr or chisel coming in contact with the ossicles. Differences between pre- and postoperative hearing levels (air- and bone-conducted) at 4000 Hz in three types of ossiculoplasty for both types of cholesteatoma are shown in Fig. 4–4. In attic cholesteatoma, there was no damage from any of the three types of ossiculoplasty: levels of air- and bone-conducted hearing were all improved after surgery. On the other hand, in adhesive cholesteatoma levels of air-conducted hearing in the group given type IV ossiculoplasties, and levels of bone-conducted hearing in groups given all three types of ossiculoplasty, became worse after surgery. The worst were those undergoing type IV ossiculoplasty: they showed a loss of 10 dB.

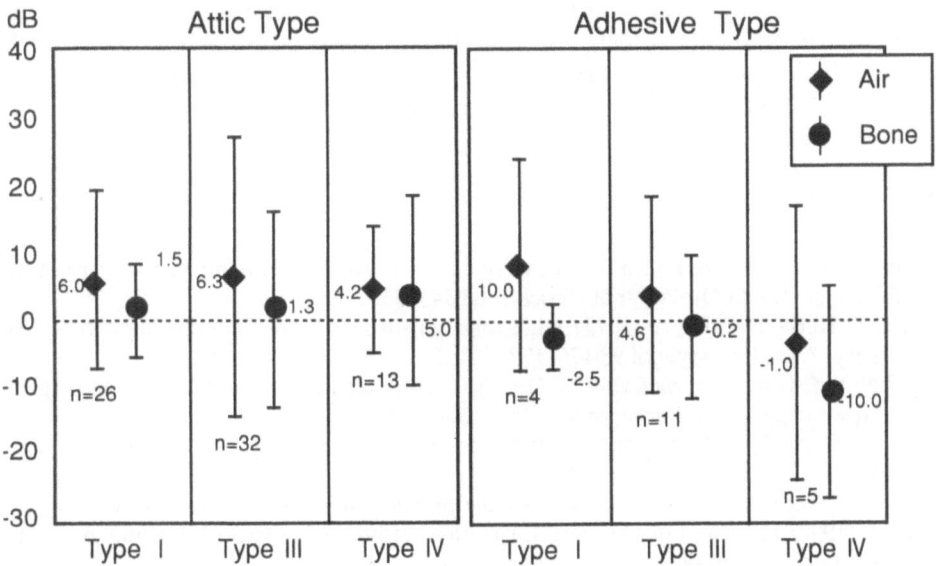

Fig. 4–4. Gains in air- (*diamonds*) and bone-conductive (*circles*) hearing at 4 KHz in each type of ossiculoplasty for attic (*left*) and adhesive (*right*) cholesteatoma

4.2.5 Discussion

Smyth (1977) reported an aggravation in thresholds for bone conduction of 10 dB through the frequencies of 500 Hz to 4000 Hz and cochlear damage from burr contact in 6% of cases undergoing canal-up procedures. Palva and co-workers (1973) reported postoperative hearing losses of high tones in the majority (82%) of those receiving radical mastoidectomy. Palmgren (1979) observed a highly significant postoperative sensorineural hearing loss of 12 dB at 4000 Hz after mastoidectomy. Ragheb and colleagues (1987) reported a mean loss of 3.5 dB at 4000 Hz. Suzuki (1983) reported postoperative hearing results in 93 ears with cholesteatoma showing an improvement of −0.2 dB in the air–bone gap after type I ossiculoplasty in 30 ears, an improvement of 7.1 dB in type III ossiculoplasty using columella in 52 ears, and an improvement of 8.4 dB in type IV ossiculoplasty using columella in 11 ears. Tos (1992) reported that 60% of 320 ears with cholesteatoma operated on using the canal-up method showed an air–bone gap within 20 dB, and 69% showed an air–bone gap within 40 dB, 2 years after surgery.

Our postoperative results showed that hearing worsened at all frequencies only for those groups receiving type III and IV ossiculoplasty for adhesive cholesteatoma. Cases with decreased bone-conducted hearing in high frequencies showed a tendency to incur damage to the inner ear during surgery, especially in adhesive cholesteatoma. In conclusion, we find anterior tympanotomy itself is not harmful to the inner ear, because no damage was seen in all types of ossiculoplasty for groups with attic cholesteatoma even though the same anterior tympanotomy was done for both types of cholesteatoma. In adhesive cholesteatoma, however, damage to bone-conducted hearing seemed to result from surgical contact directly on the stapes, which is impossible to avoid in eradication of pathological tissue in adhesive cholesteatoma, although it is possible to eliminate this danger in almost all cases of attic cholesteatoma.

References

Palmgren O (1979) Long-term results of open cavity and tympanomastoid surgery of the chronic ear. Acta Otolarygnol (Stockh) 88:343–349

Palva T, Karja T, Palva A (1973) High-tone sensorineural losses following chronic ear surgery. Arch Otolaryngol 98:176–178

Ragheb SM, Gantz BJ, McCabe BF (1987) Hearing results after cholesteatoma surgery: the Iowa experience. Laryngoscope 97:1254–1263

Smyth GDL (1977) Sensorineural hearing loss in chronic ear surgery. Ann Otol Laryngol 86:3–8

Suzuki J (1983) Approach to conductive deafness (in Japanese). Shinohara, Tokyo

Tos M (1992) Hearing after surgery for cholesteatoma using various techniques. Auris Nasus Larynx 16:61–73

Chapter 5
Surgical Findings of Anterior Tympanotomy in the Cholesteatomatous Ear

In this chapter, surgical findings in anterior tympanotomy on the tympanic diaphragm, especially on the partition attached to cholesteatoma near the supratubal recess, are explained and discussed. As cholesteatoma develops (usually in the poorly pneumatized ear), these intraoperative results can be used in place of anatomical landmarks on the tympanic diaphragm. In this study, we measured the bony partition removed during anterior tympanotomy using angled sounds with tips 3, 4, and 5 mm long. The length of the bony partition, the width of the drilled rough bony surface (indicating thickness of the bony partition at the base), and the size of the supratubal recess were measured.

5.1 Attic Cholesteatoma

The results obtained from 162 ears were analyzed. In 159 ears, the bony partition could be classified into three types: plate type, pyramidal type, and anterior type (Fig. 5–1). In three ears, classification was impossible because of incomplete surgical records.

5.1.1 Plate Type of Partition

The bony partition (anterior attic bony plate) of this type is thin and long, reaching to the malleal head with a widely developed supratubal recess (Fig. 5–1a). This type was observed in 49% of all cases of attic cholesteatoma. Its length ranged from 1 mm to 6 mm, with an average of 3 mm; its thickness ranged from 0.5 to 2.0 mm, with an average of 1.5 mm. The surgical procedure to remove this bony septum is usually easy. In some cases, the bony plate of the tensor tympani was recognizable, as was the mucosal fold of the tensor tympani, which varied in size and was with or without perforation. Removal of the tensor tympani mucosal fold must not be omitted, if it is not perforated. The bony plate of the tensor tympani must also be removed, if the opening to the eustachian tube is small. The mucosa in the supratubal recess is kept in place if it is not pathological.

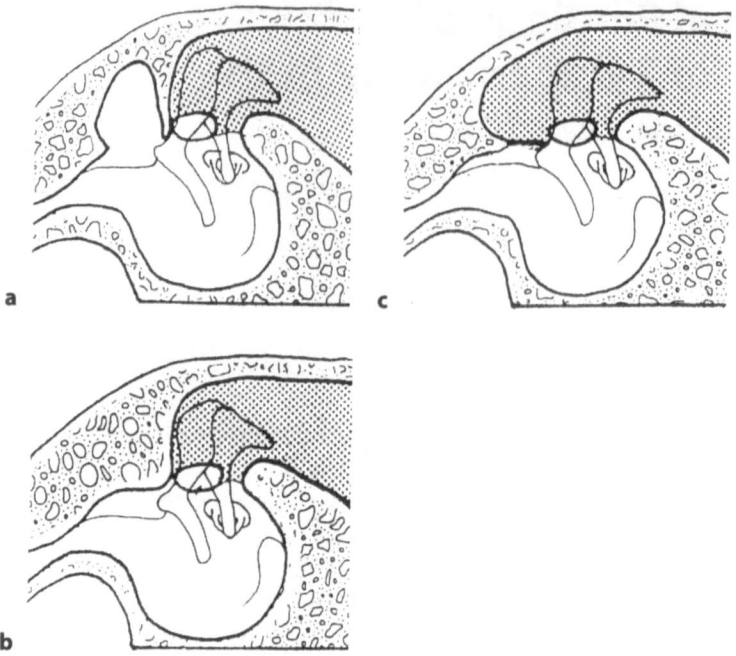

Fig. 5–1a–c. Classification of three types of supratubal partitions and incidence of each in attic cholesteatoma. **a** Plate type, 49%. **b** Pyramidal type, 28.3%. **c** Anterior type, 20.1%

TABLE 5–1. Distribution by age in years of patients with plate-type partition and recurrence in attic cholesteatoma

Age groups	~9	10–19	20–29	30–39	40–49	50–59	60+	Totals
Cases	8	16	5	10	22	14	5	80
Recurrence	2	2	1	1	1	0	0	7
Per cent (%)	25.0	12.5	20.0	10.0	4.5	0	0	8.7

Distribution by age and number of recurrences of cholesteatoma is shown in Table 5–1. The rate of recurrence is 8.7% overall, being a little more frequent in younger groups.

5.1.2 Pyramidal Type of Partition

Bony partitions of this type have a massive bony pyramidal shape with small or absent supratubal recess, as shown in Fig. 5–1b. This type was observed in 28.3% of all cases of attic cholesteatoma. In a few cases, there was a small notch at the top of the bony plate, which may be a remnant of the superior supratubal recess.

The surgical procedure to make a new ventilation route by removing this bony partition is very difficult. It is recommended to start drilling bony tissue near the anterior process of the malleus or the anterior mallear ligament. In this process,

TABLE 5–2. Distribution by age in years of patients with pyramidal-type partition and recurrence in attic cholesteatoma

Age groups	~9	10–19	20–29	30–39	40–49	50–59	60+	Totals
Cases	5	6	4	9	10	6	5	45
Recurrence	0	2	0	2	0	0	0	4
Per cent (%)	0	33.3	0	22.2	0	0	0	8.8

damage to the chorda tympani and the anterior tympanic artery must be avoided. It is useful to search for the inferior supratubal recess from the protympanum to find a route for drilling. In cases with an intact ossicular chain or good hearing, temporarily luxating the incudomalleal joint is recommended, to avoid damage to the inner ear. Mucosa on the bony partition (mucoperiosteum) must be retained for later use to cover the raw surface of the bone.

Thickness at the base of this type of plate ranged from 3 to 5 mm, and its length from 2 to 5 mm. Distribution by age and number of recurrences are shown in Table 5–2. There was no special distribution by age, although recurrence (8.8%) was more frequent in the younger generation.

5.1.3 Anterior Type of Partition

In the anterior type, cholesteatoma develops into the anterior space near the malleal head, coincident with the space for the supratubal recess (Fig. 5–1c). The cavity made at the end of removal of cholesteatoma, therefore, is coincident with the supratubal recess. The bony plate of the tensor tympani partitions the cholesteatoma from the protympanum, and the mucosal fold of the tensor tympani is located parallel to the semicanal of the tensor tympani muscle. In some cases, however, the inferior supratubal recess is recognizable through a perforated tensor tympani mucosal fold; 32 of 159 (20.1%) ears with attic cholesteatoma were classified in this group.

Measurement of bony septa in this group was almost impossible because the partition lies on a line with the visual axis. The bony plate is short, and the mucosal fold is also short and very thick. The anterior attic bony plate usually observed at the front of the malleal head is absent. Therefore, it cannot be clearly known whether the bony plate has been destroyed and absorbed by cholesteatoma. We conclude, however, from knowledge obtained in the normally

TABLE 5–3. Distribution by age in years of patients with anterior-type partition and recurrence in attic cholesteatoma

Age groups	~9	10–19	20–29	30–39	40–49	50–59	60+	Totals
Cases	8	7	1	2	5	8	3	34
Recurrence	1	1	0	1	0	0	0	3
Per cent (%)	12.5	14.3	0	50.0	0	0	0	8.8

developed ear, that the anterior attic bony plate is located anteriorly and inferiorly, and thus the superior supratubal recess has not developed in these patients. Distribution by age and number of recurrences is shown in Table 5–3. The rate of recurrence was 8.8% in younger groups.

5.2 Adhesive Cholesteatoma

In 61 cases of adhesive cholesteatoma, the partitions were classified into the following four types: plate type, pyramidal type, anterior type, and mucosal fold

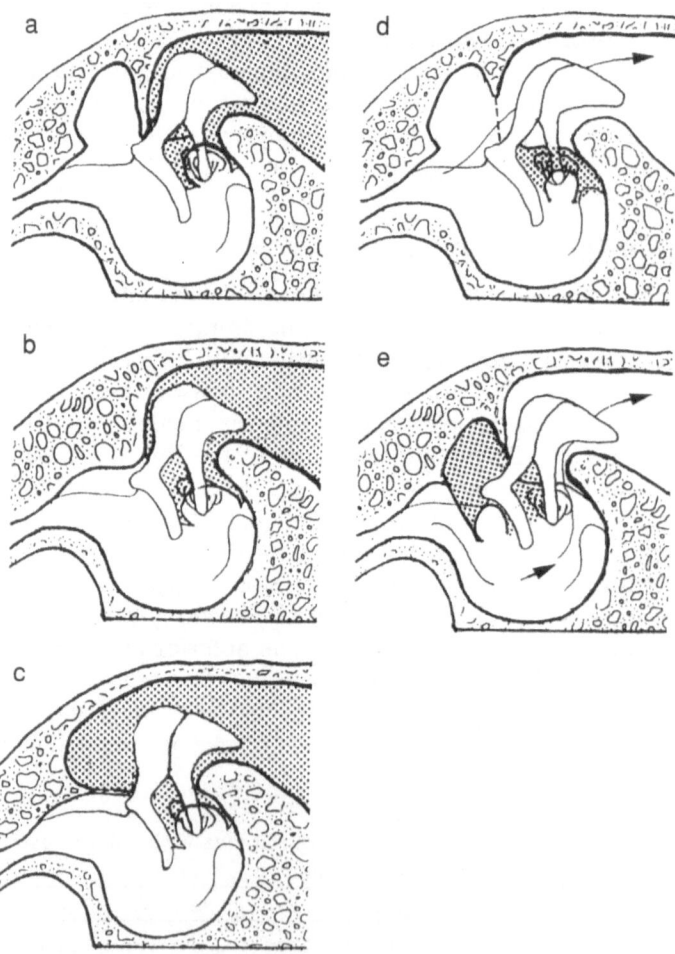

FIG. 5–2a–e. Classification of supratubal partitions and incidence of each type in adhesive cholesteatoma. **a** Plate type, 49.1%. **b** Pyramidal type, 26.3%. **c** Anterior type, 14.0%. **d** Mucosal fold type, 8.7%. **e** Tensor fold type. *Arrows* indicate open ventilator route

type (Fig. 5–2). In one special case, cholesteatoma developed into the supratubal recess from the adhered anterior superior quadrant. Four ears could not be classified because of incomplete surgical records.

5.2.1 Plate Type of Partition

The plate type is the same as that in attic cholesteatoma and was observed in 45.9% of these 61 cases. The length of the plate ranged from 2 mm to 4 mm, most frequently being 2–3 mm long in both well- and poorly pneumatized ears. The thickness ranged from 1 to 2 mm. Distribution by age and number of recurrences are shown in Table 5–4. Two cases in the age group for teens showed recurrences.

TABLE 5–4. Distribution by age in years of patients with plate-type recurrence in adhesive cholesteatoma

Age groups	~9	10–19	20–29	30–39	40–49	50–59	60+	Totals
Cases	1	7	1	5	8	5	1	28
Recurrence	0	2	0	0	0	0	0	2
Per cent (%)	0	28.6	0	0	0	0	0	7.1

5.2.2 Pyramidal Type of Partition

The pyramidal type was observed in 26.3% of all adhesive cases. Thickness at the base was about 4 mm, and length was from 2 to 3 mm. Distribution by age and number of recurrences (20%) are shown in Table 5–5.

TABLE 5–5. Distribution by age in years of patients with pyramidal-type partition and recurrence in adhesive cholesteatoma

Age groups	~9	10–19	20–29	30–39	40–49	50–59	60+	Totals
Cases	4	0	1	3	4	4	3	15
Recurrence	1	0	0	1	1	0	0	3
Per cent (%)	25.0	0	0	33.3	25.0	0	0	20.0

5.2.3 Anterior Type of Partition

The anterior type was observed in 8 (13.1%) of these 61 cases. Cholesteatoma developed from the posterior superior quadrant into the anterior malleal space under its neck or manubrium and through the isthmus into the epitympanum.

TABLE 5–6. Distribution by age in years of patients with anterior-type partition and recurrence in adhesive cholesteatoma

Age groups	~9	10–19	20–29	30–39	40–49	50–59	60+	Totals
Cases	0	0	0	1	4	3	0	8
Recurrence	0	0	0	0	0	0	0	0
Per cent (%)	0	0	0	0	0	0	0	0

The tympanic aperture of the eustachian tube was closed by adhered eardrum. In two ears, a small bony plate was recognized at the tegmen tympani. It is, however, not clear whether that bony plate was the anterior attic bony plate absorbed by cholesteatoma. Distribution by age is shown in Table 5–6. This type of partition was observed only in middle-aged groups. There was no case of recurrence in this group.

5.2.4 Mucosal Fold Type of Partition

In this type, cholesteatoma developed from the posterior superior quadrant of an adhered eardrum and localized only near the oval window or the sinus tympani. The mucosal fold type is found only in adhesive cholesteatoma and is called precholesteatoma by some otosurgeons. The anterior attic bony plate in five ears (8.7%) was short, and the mucosal folds were perforated, making a ventilation route into the epitympanum as in a pneumatized ear. The tympanic isthmus was closed completely by the retracted ossicles. There was, therefore, no route into the epitympanum and also no negative pressure, whch drove the cholesteatoma to develop into the epitympanum.

In one ear (1.7%) in the group of teens, cholesteatoma developed from the adhered anterior superior quadrant into the supratubal recess. In this case, the long anterior attic bony plate with a short mucosal fold and the intact tensor tympani mucosal fold closed off the supratubal recess from both the epitympanum and the protympanum. A ventilation route was patent, however, from the eustachian tube through the hypotympanum and the posterior tympanic isthmus, so we gave this type a temporary name, the tensor fold type. Distribution of this type of partition by age is shown in Table 5–7.

TABLE 5–7. Distribution by age in years of patients with mucoasal fold-type partition and recurrence in adhesive cholesteatoma

Age groups	~9	10–19	20–29	30–39	40–49	50–59	60+	Totals
Cases	2	1	0	0	0	3	0	6
Recurrence	0	0	0	0	0	0	0	0
Per cent (%)	0	0	0	0	0	0	0	0

5.3 Pathological Development of the Supratubal Recess

In Chapter 2, the developmental process of the supratubal recess from embryo to fetus to child to adult in the well-pneumatized ear was described. In this chapter, the supratubal recess in the poorly pneumatized ear is reported, as observed in cholesteatomatous ears. We thus have covered the developmental process of the anterior tympanic diaphragm in both well- and poorly pneumatized ears throughout the human life span.

The supratubal recess does not exist in the human embryo or fetus. It begins to develop gradually in late fetal life and rapidly after birth, in parallel with age and otologic pneumatization. If development of the saccus medius and anticus is normal, the bony plate (anterior attic bony plate) between the sacs becomes shorter and thinner, changing to the anterior attic mucosal fold, which further becomes thinner and often perforates to communicate with surrounding spaces. The bony plate between the labyrinthine and tympanic branches of the saccus

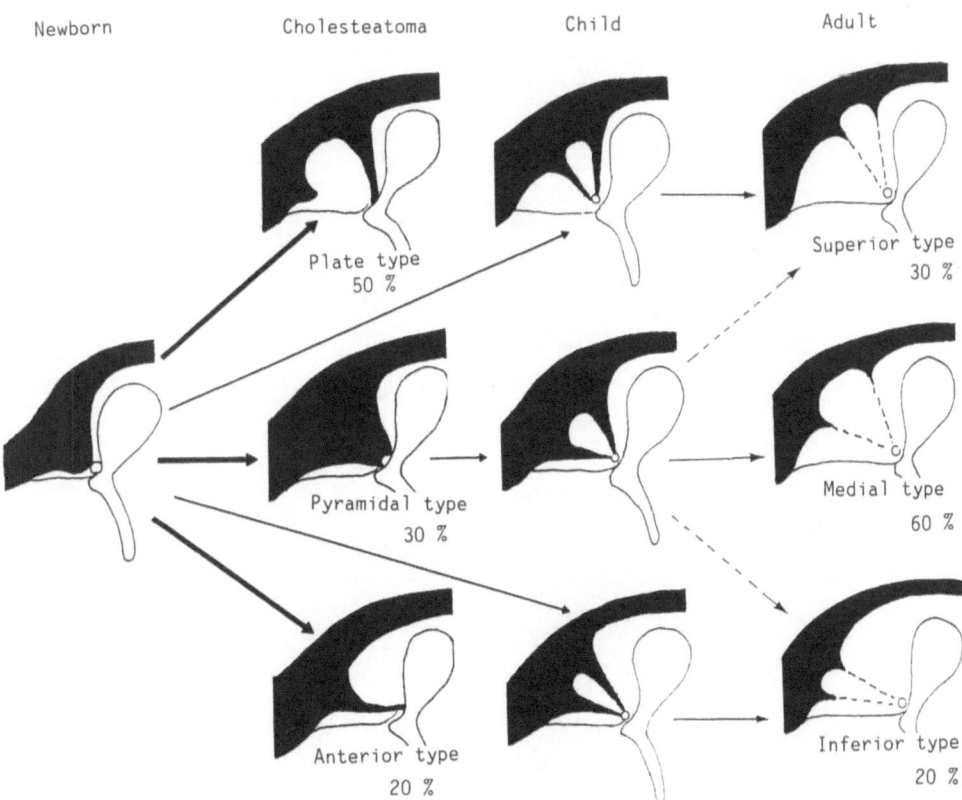

FIG. 5–3. Normal and pathological developmental process of area of the supratubal recess from birth to adulthood

anticus (tensor tympani bony plate) undergoes the same process as the anterior attic bony plate, transforming into the tensor tympani mucosal fold.

If pneumatization is stopped directly after birth, the bony portion in the supratubal area leads to a pyramidal type of bony partition. If pneumatization progresses further and the recess develops more emphatically from the protympanum (saccus anticus), then it leads to the superior type of supratubal recess found in well-pneumatized ears and to the type of plate found in poorly pneumatized cholesteatomatous ears. If pneumatization from the epitympanum (saccus medius) is more marked, it leads to the inferior type of supratubal recess found in well-pneumatized ears and to the anterior type of plate found in poorly pneumatized cholesteatomatous ears. Developmental processes in the supratubal recess from birth to the adult stage in well- and poorly pneumatized ears are explained in the schematic flowchart shown in Fig. 5–3.

Chapter 6
Computed Tomography of the Cholesteatomatous Ear

The temporal bone comprises five parts: (1) a squamous portion, (2) a petrous portion, (3) a tympanic portion, (4) a mastoid portion, and (5) a styloid portion. The petrous portion is the most important in radiology for cholesteatoma; it houses all of the inner ear, the epitympanic cavity, and the supratubal recess in the protympanum. Anterolaterally the petrous connects with the the tympanic portion at the petrotympanic fissure (Glaserian fissure), which forms the passage for the chorda tympani and the anterior tympanic artery. Posteriorly, it connects with the squamous portion at the petrosquamous suture, which remains as Koerner's septum, projecting into the superior portion of the mastoid antrum to form a surgical landmark.

In computed tomography (CT) of the cholesteatomatous ear, the following points must be identified and evaluated in addition to the inner ear and the internal auditory meatus: the tuba auditiva, the semicanal of the tensor tympani muscle, the tensor tympani tendon, peritubal air cells, the supratubal recess, the anterior attic bony plate (anterior attic mucosal fold), the malleus, incus, and stapes, the geniculate ganglion, the facial nerve, and the tympanic isthmus (Fig. 6–1). The CT scanner we used was the GE-T-8800 (Milwaukee, WI, USA), which scans thicknesses of 1.0 mm at intervals every other millimeter. The head is inclined at a 30° angle from the orbitomeatal line (semiaxial), to avoid irradiating the eyes and to obtain precise evaluation of the eustachian tube. In this chapter, a semiaxial CT scan of temporal bones as if sectioned through the geniculate ganglion and one or two "slices" from lower sections are shown in the figures that follow; the supratubal recess, anterior attic bony plate, and ossicles can be observed most clearly in one section.

6.1 Computed Tomographic Scan of Normal Temporal Bone

Figure 6–2 shows normal temporal bone. A typical supratubal recess is shown in Fig. 6–2a, in which the well-developed and well-ventilated supratubal recess (R) is visible in front of the malleal head. The posterior borderline is the anterior attic bony plate (P). The geniculate ganglion (G) is visible at the labyrinthine side of

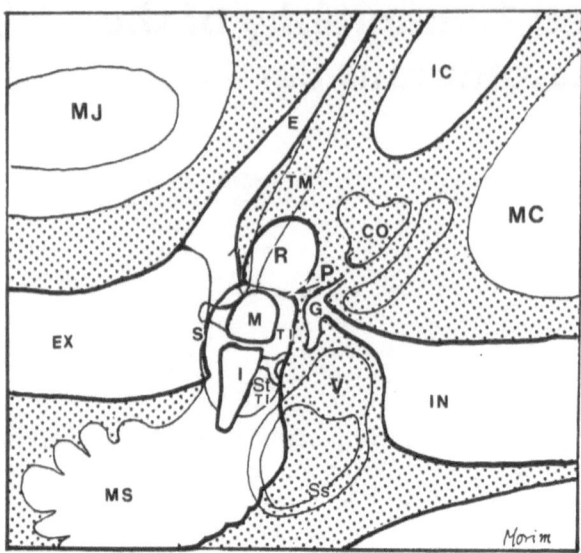

Fig. 6–1. Radiological anatomy of the temporal bone. Several slices from the tympanic tegmen to the stapes are superimposed into one slice. *R*, supratubal recess; *P*, anterior attic bony plate; *G*, geniculate ganglion; *M*, malleus; *I*, incus; *St*, stapes; *TI*, tympanic isthmus; *S*, scutum; *V*, vestibulum; *CO*, cochlea; *Ss*, semicircular canal; *E*, eustachian tube; *TM*, tensor tympani semicanal; *EX*, external ear canal; *IN*, internal ear canal; *MS*, mastoid air cells; *MC*, middle cranial fossa; *MJ*, mandibular joint; *IC*, internal carotid artery

the supratubal recess. Well-developed mastoid air cells and Koerner's septum (K) are recognizable in the center. The internal auditory meatus (I) is not pathological.

Figure 6–2b, showing a small supratubal recess, is a section sliced more inferiorly than the section through the geniculate ganglion. The supratubal recess (R) is small, although it usually becomes larger in lower sections. The anterior attic bony plate (P) is rudimentary, and its mucosal fold is probably perforated. The tympanic isthmus (T) is open wide. Between the internal carotid artery (CA) and the recess, the semicanal (S) of the tensor tympani is visible.

In the ear shown in Fig. 6–2c, the large supratubal recess (R) is larger than the epitympanic space containing the ossicles (O). The bony plate (P) is rudimentary, and there is no septum closing off the recess. The mastoid cavity is aerated very well.

In Fig. 6–2d, the air cell-shaped supratubal recess (R) is rather small and air cells (arrows) have developed around the recess. Histological study showed no communication between the supratubal recess and air cells, but this is not clearly visible in the CT scan. (See classifications of supratubal recesses in Chapter 2.)

Fig. 6–2a–d. Computed tomography (CT) scan of normal temporal bone.

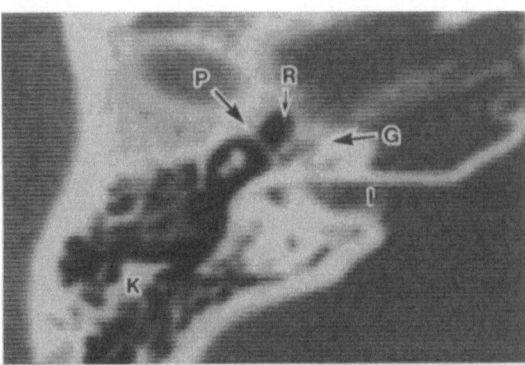

a Typical supratubal recess at the level of the geniculate ganglion. *R*, supratubal recess; *P*, anterior attic bony plate; *G*, geniculate ganglion; *I*, internal auditory canal; *K*, Koerner's septum

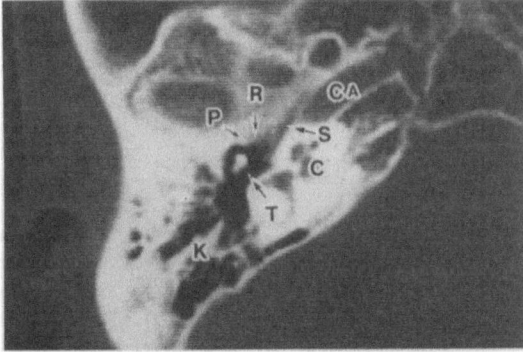

b Small supratubal recess sliced at lower level. *R*, supratubal recess; *P*, anterior attic bony plate; *T*, tympanic isthmus; *S*, tensor tympani semicanal; *C*, cochlea; *CA*, carotid artery; *K*, Koerner's septum

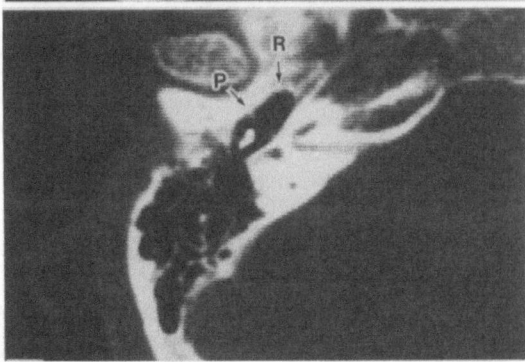

c Large supratubal recess. *R*, supratubal recess; *P*, rudimentary anterior attic bony plate

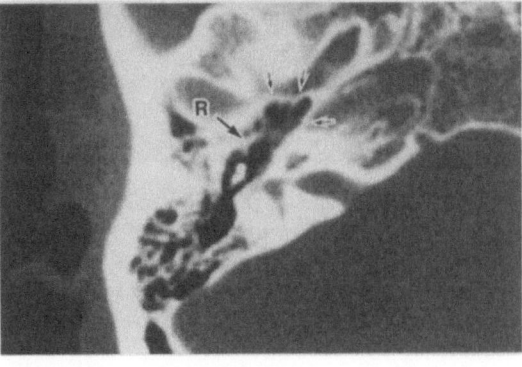

d Air cell-shaped supratubal recess. *R*, supratubal recess; *arrows*, air cells around the supratubal recess

6.2 Computed Tomographic Scan of Attic Cholesteatoma

Our most important question was whether differentiation of the bony partition (into the three types reported in Chapter 5) is possible, using CT. Figures 6–3 to 6–5 show the bony partitions of each of the three types—plate type, pyramidal type, and anterior type—as confirmed by intraoperative observations.

6.2.1 Plate Type of Partition in Attic Cholesteatoma

Figure 6–3 demonstrates the plate type of bony partition in a 14-year-old boy. The supratubal recess (R) is filled with air and distinctly bordered by a soft tissue mass (cholesteatoma) in the epitympanum and the mastoid antrum. The partition

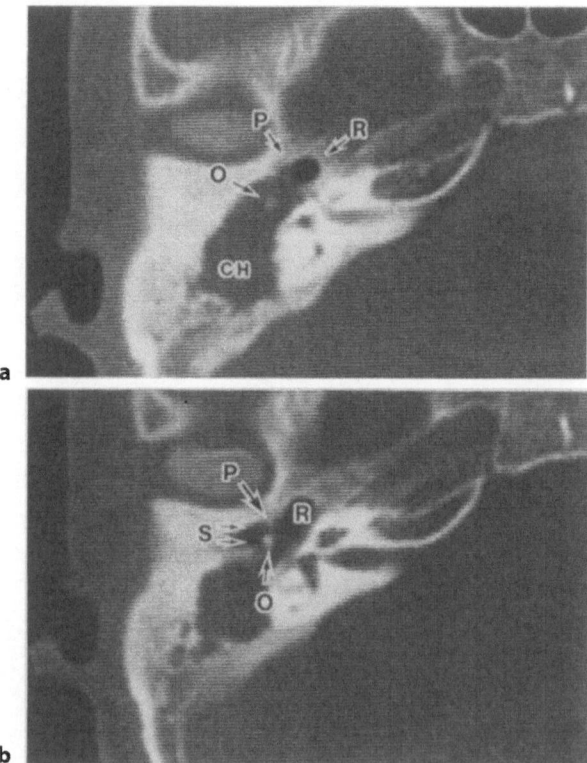

FIG. 6–3a,b. Plate type of partition in attic cholesteatoma. **a** Plate type of partition in a 14-year-old boy. *R*, supratubal recess; *P*, plate type of partition (anterior attic bony plate); *O*, carious malleus; *CH*, cholesteatoma. **b** Plate type of partition, one slice lower than the section of Fig. 6–3a. *Two small arrows* indicate erosion of the scutum. *R*, supratubal recess; *P*, plate type of partition (anterior attic bony plate); *O*, carious malleus; *S*, eroded scutum

between them is not clearly a bony plate, but is of the "plate type," which was confirmed intraoperatively. The ossicles (O) are pitted with decay.

Figure 6–3b shows a section one slice lower than in Fig. 6–3a. The small arrows (S) indicate erosion of the scutum by cholesteatoma. The recess (R) is elongated anteriorly, connecting to the eustachian tube. This plate-type partition (P) is so thin that it is not clear whether it is bony or membranous because of the "partial volume" effect.

6.2.2 Pyramidal Type of Partition in Attic Cholesteatoma

Figure 6–4a shows the pyramidal type of partition, sliced at the level of the geniculate ganglion, as observed in a 12-year-old boy. The supratubal recess is not visible in front of the eroded malleus. The thick bony area (P) is a pyramidal type of bony partition. The geniculate ganglion (G) is clearly recognizable. The scutum (S) is widely eroded, and the incudal head has disappeared.

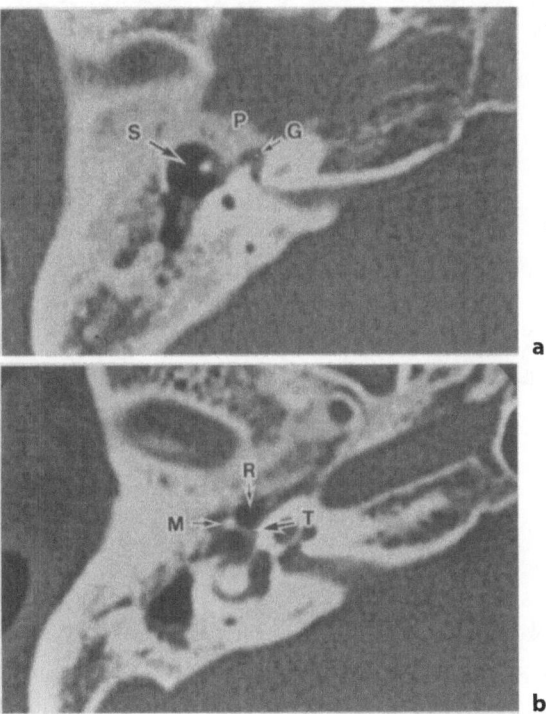

FIG. 6–4a–d. Pyramidal type of partition in attic cholesteatoma. a Pyramidal type of partition sliced at the level of the geniculate ganglion in a 12-year-old boy. P, pyramidal type of partition; G, geniculate ganglion; S, eroded scutum. b Pyramidal type of partition, two slices lower than the section of Fig. 6–4a. R, inferior supratubal recess; M, mallear neck; T, tensor tympani tendon

Figure 6–4b shows a section two slices lower than in Fig. 6–4a. The supratubal recess (lower supratubal recess) is visible. It is well aerated and borders posteriorly on the tympanic isthmus, demarcated by the tensor tympani tendon (T), which attaches to the neck of the malleus (M).

Figure 6–4c shows a second case of the pyramidal type of partition, seen in a 10-year-old boy. There is a thick bony partition (P) between the epitympanum and the small supratubal recess (R). This recess disappears one slice up. In the attic and mastoid, cholesteatoma is visible.

Figure 6–4d shows a section one slice lower than in Fig. 6–4c. The bony plate (P) becomes thinner in this section as the supratubal recess becomes larger. The semicanal of the tensor tympani muscle (M) is visible. The pyramidal type of bony partition in this second case is thinner than in the first case.

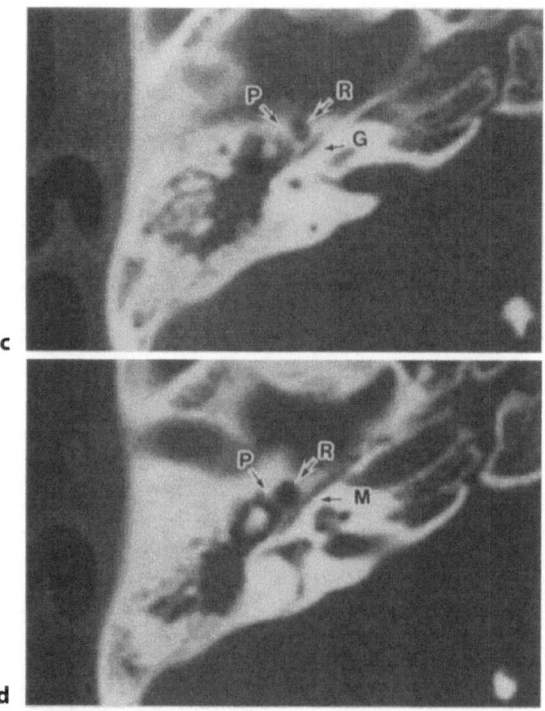

Fig. 6–4. (*Continued.*) **c** Thinner pyramidal type of partition, in a 10-year-old boy. *R*, supratubal recess; *P*, pyramidal type of partition (thick anterior attic bony plate); *G*, geniculate ganglion. **d** Thinner pyramidal type of partiton, one slice lower than the section of Fig. 6–4c. *R*, inferior supratubal recess; *P*, pyramidal type of partition; *M*, tensor tympani muscle

6.2.3 Anterior Type of Partition in Attic Cholesteatoma

Figure 6–5a shows the anterior type of partition, observed in an 11-year-old girl. No partition is seen at the usual position. Cholesteatoma (C) has developed into the supratubal recess (R), although no dense mass of soft tissue is seen in this area because it was removed before the CT examination. A cholesteatomatous mass is visible in the mastoid cavity. No ossicles are visible.

Figure 6–5b shows a section one slice lower than Fig. 6–5a. The supratubal recess (R) and the scutum (S) are expanded (arrows), and the eustachian tube (E) is filled with dense soft tissue, which indicates retention of mucus because of tubal dysfunction. The partition is not visible because it is located parallel to the plane of the CT scan.

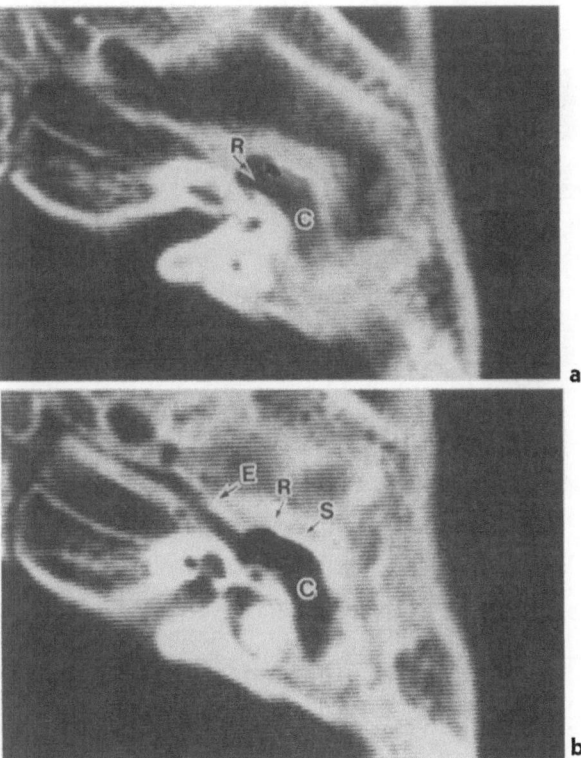

Fig. 6–5a,b. Anterior type of partition in attic cholesteatoma. **a** CT scan shows no partition at usual position. *R*, supratubal area covered with cholesteatomatous matrix; *C*, cholesteatomatous debris. **b** One slice lower than the section in Fig. 6–5a. *E*, eustachian tube; *R*, supratubal recess; *S*, eroded scutum

6.3 Illustration of Bony Partitions in Attic Cholesteatoma

Figure 6–6 shows sections through the geniculate ganglion. The ossicles, normally shaped, are also shown.

6.3.1 Plate Type of Partition in Attic Cholesteatoma

A sharp borderline is seen between the supratubal recess and the epitympanum filled with cholesteatoma in Fig. 6–6a. In almost all cases, the bony plate itself, however, is not clear because of the partial volume effect. The scutum is absorbed by cholesteatoma. The ossicles are pressed against the inner ear, and the tympanic isthmus is closed.

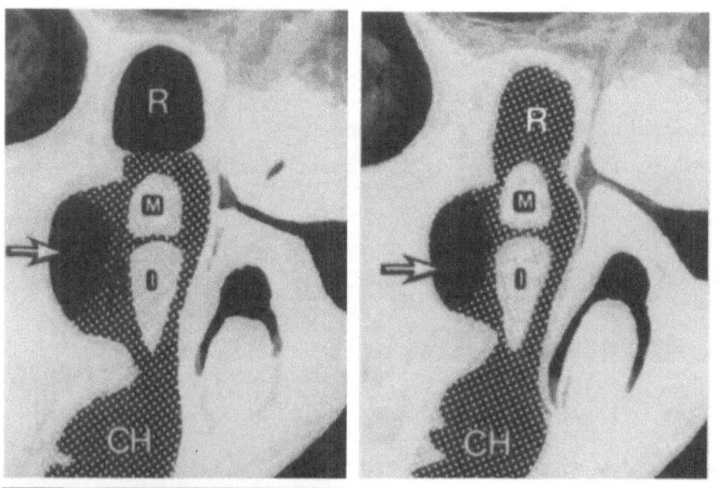

a

c

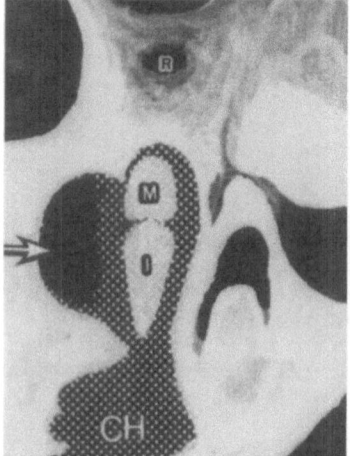

b

FIG. 6–6a–c. Partition of attic cholesteatoma in CT scan through the geniculate ganglion. **a** Plate type of partition. *R*, supratubal recess; *M*, malleus; *I*, incus; *CH*, cholesteatoma; *arrow*, eroded scutum. **b** Pyramidal type of partition. *R*, small recess; *M*, malleus; *I*, incus; *CH*, cholesteatoma. **c** Anterior type of partition. *R*, recess filled with cholesteatoma; *M*, malleus; *I*, incus; *CH*, cholesteatoma

6.3.2 Pyramidal Type of Partition in Attic Cholesteatoma

The supratubal recess cannot be recognized in front of the head of the malleus in Fig. 6–6b. The area for the recess is bony tissue here, but in lower CT sections or in some cases with thinner pyramidal bony partitions, a small recess may be visible, with a thick bony partition (as shown in this figure). Other findings are the same as those in the plate type of partition.

6.3.3 Anterior Type of Partition in Attic Cholesteatoma

The area of the supratubal recess is filled with a dense soft tissue mass, the debris of cholesteatoma (Fig. 6–6c). The partition cannot be recognized in this section through the geniculate ganglion. In lower CT sections, the eustachian tube or the inferior supratubal recess becomes visible.

6.4 Computed Tomographic Scan of Adhesive Cholesteatoma

In adhesive cholesteatoma, the partition between the epitympanum and the supratubal recess can be classified into four types: plate type, pyramidal type, anterior type, and mucosal fold type.

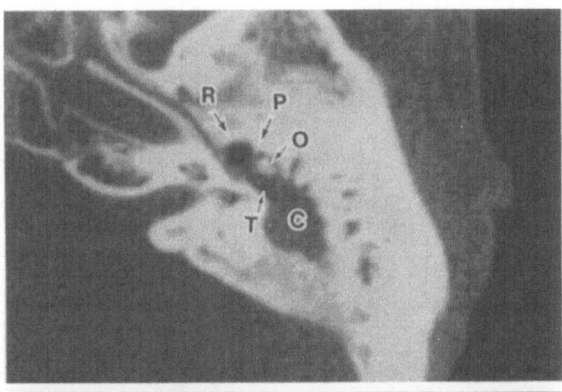

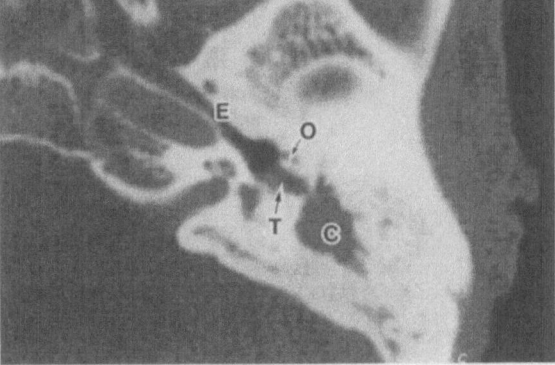

FIG. 6–7a,b. Plate type of partition in adhesive cholesteatoma. a Plate type of partition observed in a 43-year-old man. R, supratubal recess; P, anterior attic bony plate; T, tympanic isthmus; C, cholesteatoma; O, ossicle. b One slice lower than the section in Fig. 6–7a. E, eustachian tube; O, ossicle; T, tympanic isthmus; C, cholesteatoma

6.4.1 Plate Type of Partition in Adhesive Cholesteatoma

The plate type of partition was observed in a 43-year-old man (Fig. 6–7a). The supratubal recess (R) is relatively large and is filled with air. There is a clear border with the epitympanum, although no bony line is visible except its outer root. It was, however, confirmed intraoperatively that this partition was of the plate type (P). Cholesteatoma (C) has developed through the open tympanic isthmus (T), so that the ossicle (O) is pressed against the intact scutum, and the tympanic isthmus is widened.

The section shown in Fig. 6–7b is one slice lower than in Fig. 6–7a. The eustachian tube (E), the protympanum, and the supratubal recess are well aerated. There is a borderline with the epitympanum, although the bony plate is not visible. The ossicles (O) adhere to the scutum. Cholesteatoma (C) fills the widened tympanic isthmus and also the mastoid antrum.

6.4.2 Pyramidal Type of Partition in Adhesive Cholesteatoma

Figure 6–8a shows the pyramidal type of partition, observed in a 44-year-old woman. The supratubal recess (R) is small, and the bony partition (P) is thick,

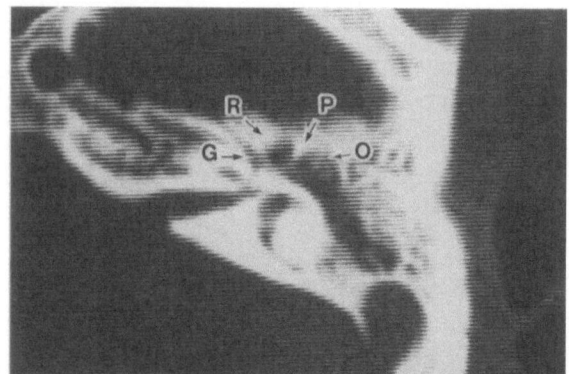

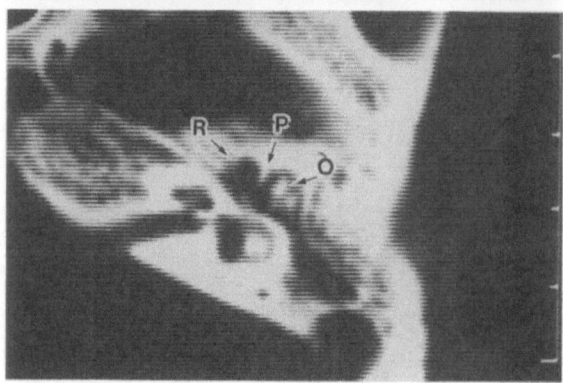

Fig. 6–8a,b. Pyramidal type of partition in adhesive cholesteatoma. **a** Pyramidal type of partition seen in a 44-year-old woman. *R*, supratubal recess; *P*, pyramidal type of bony plate; *G*, geniculate ganglion; *O*, ossicle. **b** One slice lower than the section in Fig. 6–8a. *R*, supratubal recess; *P*, pyramidal type of partition; *O*, ossicles

especially its outer side. The ossicles (O) are pressed against the scutum, and the tympanic isthmus is widened by cholesteatoma.

The section shown in Fig. 6–8b is one slice lower than in Fig. 6–8a. The supratubal recess (R) becomes larger and well ventilated. The pyramidal bony partition (P) becomes thinner in this section. The ossicles (O) are maintained well.

6.4.3 Anterior Type of Partition in Adhesive Cholesteatoma

The anterior type of partition was observed in a 43-year-old man (Fig. 6–9a). The cholesteatoma (C) is expansive and fills completely the supratubal recess (R), the epitympanum, and the mastoid cavity. Neither the anterior attic bony plate nor the ossicles are visible.

The section shown in Fig. 6–9b is two slices lower than in Fig. 6–9a. The tympanic orifice (TO) of the eustachian tube is closed by a dense mass of soft tissue, although the pharyngeal side of the eustachian tube (E) is open. This mass was a granuloma, and the partition was the thick tensor tympani mucosal fold, confirmed intraoperatively.

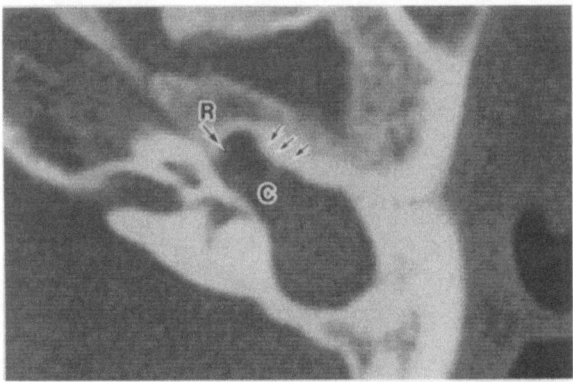

a

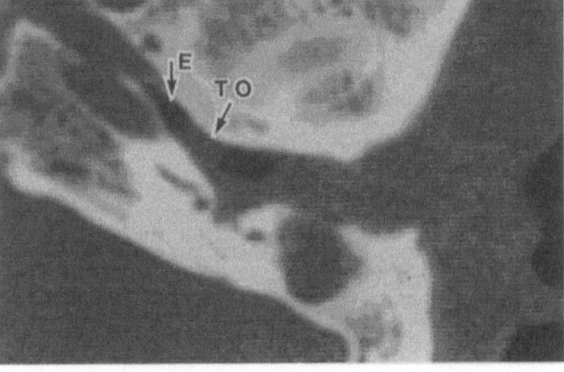

b

Fɪɢ. **6–9a,b.** Anterior type of partition in adhesive cholesteatoma. **a** Anterior type of partition seen in a 43-year-old man. *R*, recess filled with cholesteatoma; *C*, cholesteatoma. *Arrows* indicate eroded lateral wall of the recess. **b** Two slices lower than the section in Fig. 6–9a. *E*, eustachian tube; *TO*, tympanic orifice of eustachian tube, with granuloma

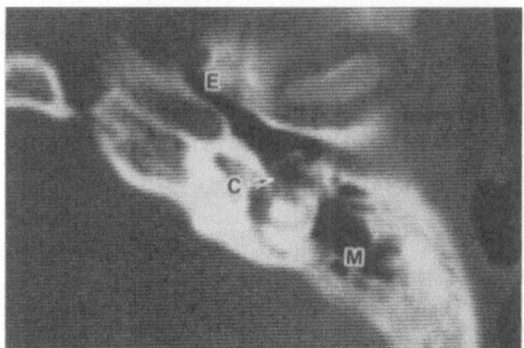

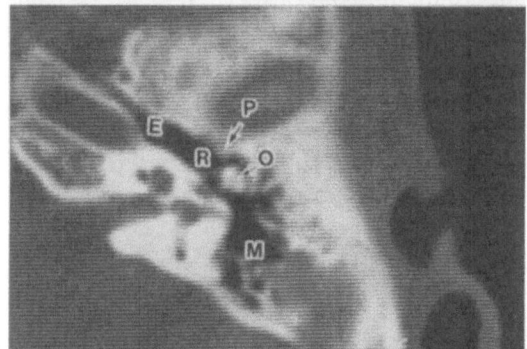

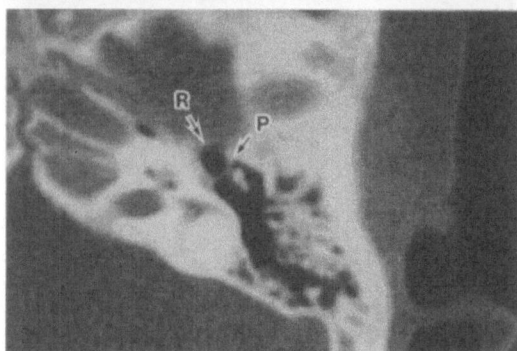

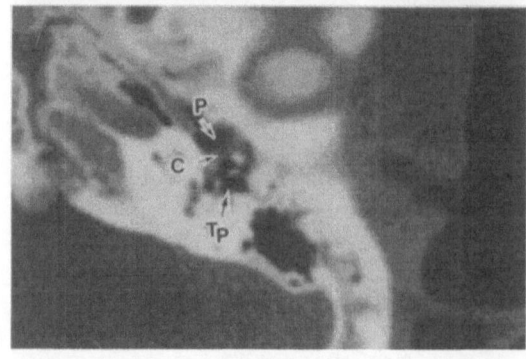

Fig. 6-10a-d. "Mucosal fold" type of partition in adhesive cholesteatoma. **a** Mucosal fold type of partition with cholesteatoma in the tympanic sinus (posterior superior quadrant [PSQ] type). *E,* eustachian tube; *C,* cholesteatoma in the tympanic sinus; *M,* mastoid with air. **b** Two slices higher than the section in Fig. 6-10a. *E,* eustachian tube; *R,* supratubal recess; *P,* mucosal fold perforated; *O,* ossicle; *M,* mastoid cells with air. **c** Mucosal fold type of partition, with cholesteatoma between the mucosal fold and the malleus (anterior superior quadrant [ASQ] type). *R,* supratubal recess; *P,* anterioir attic bony plate; *T,* tympanic isthmus; *C,* cholesteatoma. **d** One slice lower than the section in Fig. 6-10c. *E,* eustachian tube; *P,* partition; *Tp,* posterior tympanic isthmus

6.4.4 Mucosal Fold Type of Partition in Adhesive Cholesteatoma

Figure 6–10a shows the section through the oval window. Cholesteatoma (C) has developed from the posterior superior quadrant of the adhered eardrum and is located only in the tympanic sinus and near the oval window. In the mastoid cavity (M) and the eustachian tube (E), there is no pathological tissue. These findings indicate that a ventilating route is patent (through the supratubal recess to the mastoid) and that the anterior attic partition is a perforated mucosal fold. These findings were confirmed intraoperatively.

Figure 6–10b shows two slices from the upper section of Fig. 6–10a. The mastoid (M), the epitympanum, the eustachian tube (E), and the supratubal recess (R) are all well aerated without pathological changes. The anterior attic bony plate (P) is visible as a small notch at the anterior tympanic spine, and the partition is not closed. The normal ossicles (O) are positioned in the center of the epitympanum.

In Fig. 6–10c, a small cholesteatoma is visible at the anterior mallear ligament. It has developed from the anterior superior quadrant of the adhered eardrum into the epitympanum under the malleus. The plate type of partition (P) and the well-aerated supratubal recess (R) are clearly visible. The ossicles are pressed slightly toward the scutum. The tympanic isthmus is open, and the mastoid cavity is well aerated.

The section shown in Fig. 6–10d is one slice lower than in Fig. 6–10c. A small cholesteatoma (C) is recognizable between the malleus and the anterior attic partition as a dense mass of soft tissue. The posterior tympanic isthmus (Tp) is open, which explains the good aeration in this mastoid cavity. In this case, intraoperative findings completely confirmed the radiological observations.

6.5 Illustrations of Types of Bony Partitions in Adhesive Cholesteatoma

In the plate type of partition (Fig. 6–11a), a plate makes a sharp borderline between the supratubal recess and the epitympanum. The bony plate itself is difficult to distingish in almost all cases. The ossicles are pressed against the intact scutum. The tympanic isthmus is widened by cholesteatoma developed from the tympanic sinus or from near the oval window through the tympanic isthmuses.

In the pyramidal type of partition (Fig. 6–11b), the supratubal recess typically cannot be observed in front of the head of the malleus. In some cases with thinner pyramidal partitions, however, a small supratubal recess is recognizable, sandwiched off from the attic by a thick bony partition. The tympanic isthmus here is widened by cholesteatoma, and thus the ossicles are pressed against the scutum.

In the mucosal fold type of partition (Fig. 6–11c), cholesteatoma develops, usually from the posterior superior quadrant of an adhered eardrum, and localizes near the oval window or the tympanic sinus. Cholesteatoma is, therefore, visible in a section through the stapes. Aeration of the mastoid is visible in almost

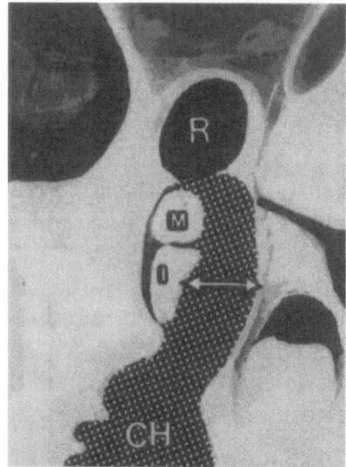

a

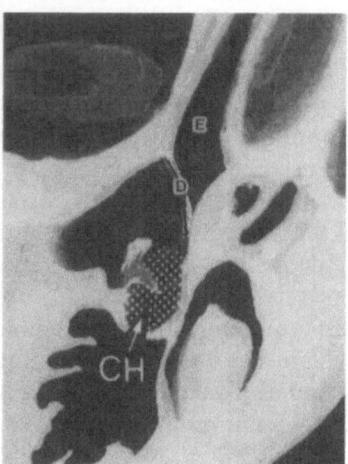

c

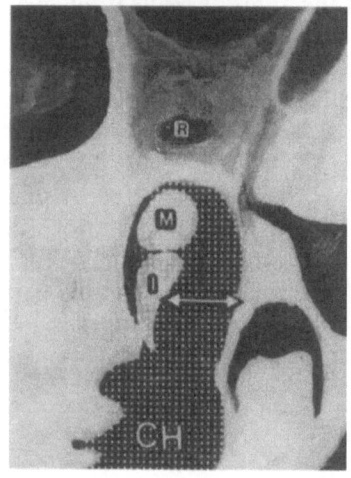

b

Fig. 6–11a–c. Illustration of partitions in adhesive cholesteatoma. **a** Plate type of partition in adhesive cholesteatoma. *R*, supratubal recess; *M*, malleus; *I*, incus; *CH*, cholesteatoma; *double-headed arrow*, tympanic isthmus widened by cholesteatoma. **b** Pyramidal type of partition in adhesive cholesteatoma. *R*, small supratubal recess in some cases. **c** Mucosal fold type of partition in adhesive cholesteatoma. *E*, eustachian tube; *D*, adhered eardrum; *CH*, cholesteatoma in the tympanic sinus

all cases. In a section as seen through the geniculate ganglion, the supratubal recess is well developed without the bony partition that closes the ventilating route from the epitympanum. In "posterior cases," cholesteatoma develops from the adhered anterior superior quadrant and localizes under the malleus or in the superior supratubal recess. In any case, one ventilation route at least is open among the three ventilation routes: by the supratubal recess, or by the anterior or posterior tympanic isthmus.

Current developments in CT radiography are dramatic: we can now see three-dimensional reconstructions or helical scans. Furthermore, magnetic resonance imaging (MRI) has made it possible to differentiate dense masses of soft tissue seen in CT scans as cholesteatoma, cholesterin granuloma, simple granuloma, or several kinds of cysts or tumors. Full discussion of these new areas must, however, be omitted from this book.

Chapter 7
Pathogenesis of Cholesteatoma

There are several different theories that attempt to explain the etiology of cholesteatoma. The three most popular original theories are (1) the retraction pocket theory states that cholesteatoma forms by accumulation of debris in retraction pockets arising from Shrapnell's membrane or from the adhered pars tensa, caused by occlusion of the eustachian tube (Bezold 1908); (2) the migration theory states that squamous epithelium which has migrated into the middle ear through a perforated tympanic membrane proliferates there (Habermann 1889); and (3) the metaplastic theory states that squamous metaplasia of the middle ear mucosa forms following chronic inflammation (Wendt 1873).

Since the introduction of these theories, numerous papers have appeared supporting or criticizing each of them. However, we have never experienced even one case in which the pathogenesis can be presumed to have occurred by one of the mechanisms of the latter two theories. On the other hand, almost all our cases of primary or recurrent cholesteatoma show no contradiction with the first, the retraction pocket theory. Therefore, in this chapter our discussion is confined to retraction cholesteatomas caused by probable negative pressure in the epitympanum.

7.1 Negative Pressure in the Epitympanum Caused by an Osseous Tympanic Diaphragm

The tympanic diaphragm is a septum between the mesotympanum and the epitympanum. This diaphragm is composed of a bony plate and many mucosal folds with a passage. The normal middle ear has a tympanic diaphragm constituted mainly of mucosal folds. I named this type of diaphragm the membranous tympanic diaphragm. On the other hand, the cholesteatoma ear has a large bony plate without a passage, so I named this type the osseous tympanic diaphragm. Figure 2–3 (see Chapter 2) illustrates the tympanic diaphragm (looking from the tegmen tympani), as reported by Proctor (1989). He did not, however, precisely illustrate the area of the supratubal recess.

Figure 7–1a is our modified illustration of the tympanic diaphragm in a well-pneumatized ear, in which ventilation is possible through the supratubal recess from the protympanum to the attic as well as by the route through the tympanic isthmuses, as discussed in Chapter 2. Under these conditions, negative pressure cannot develop in the epitympanum even when the tympanic isthmuses are closed. In an ear with such a tympanic diaphragm, there is no possibility of developing retraction of Shrapnell's membrane. I would like to propose that this type of diaphragm be named the membranous tympanic diaphragm.

Figure 7–1b shows the bony or osseous tympanic diaphragm observed in the cholesteatomatous ear, i.e., the poorly pneumatized ear, in which ventilation of the epitympanum is possible only through the tympanic isthmuses. Negative pressure can therefore develop, localizing in the epitympanum, and thus only Shrapnell's membrane retracts into the epitympanum when both anterior and posterior tympanic isthmuses are closed. In an ear with adhesions of the pars tensa, the posterior superior quadrant of the eardrum retracts into the epitympanum through the posterior tympanic isthmus when the anterior tympanic isthmus is closed, regardless of tubal occlusion or patency.

Wittmaack (1933) stated that persistence of hyperplastic embryonic mucoperiosteum in the attic might cause adhesions to form pockets in various

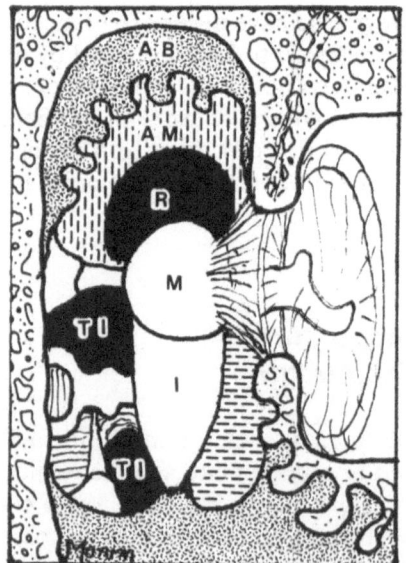 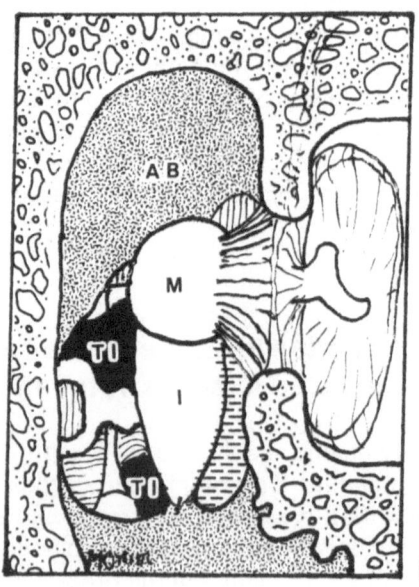

Fig. 7–1a,b. Tympanic diaphragm viewed from the tympanic tegmen. **a** Membranous tympanic diaphragm in well-pneumatized ear. **b** Osseous tympanic diaphragm in cholesteatomatous ear. *AB*, anterior attic bony plate; *AM*, anterior attic mucosal fold; *M*, malleus; *I*, incus; *TI*, tympanic isthmus; *R*, supratubal recess

portions in the attic with the resultant "attic bloc," and that these might further cause an arrest in pneumatization of the temporal bone, thus accounting for the high frequency with which retraction cholesteatomas are seen in poorly pneumatized ears. The bony tympanic diaphragm is a consequence of poor pneumatization of the temporal bone. In the next section, we discuss pneumatization in cholesteatoma and other pathological ears.

7.2 Pneumatization in Cholesteatoma and in Other Diseases of the Middle Ear

In 1989 we did comparative studies of pneumatization in cholesteatomatous ears and in other pathological conditions in the middle ear. Our materials were Schuller's x-ray photographs of 101 ears with attic and adhesive cholesteatomas, 261 with chronic otitis media, 39 with adhesive otitis media, 234 with otitis media with effusion, and 126 normal ears. The size of the pneumatized area was measured precisely with a planimeter (Miyanaga and Morimutsu 1989). Figure 7–2 shows the area of pneumatized air cells in normal temporal bone at 5-year intervals. The pneumatization stops developing at age 15, and thereafter it stays roughly the same size. This means that a predisposition to development of cholesteatoma in the temporal bone is formed in childhood up to the age of 15 years.

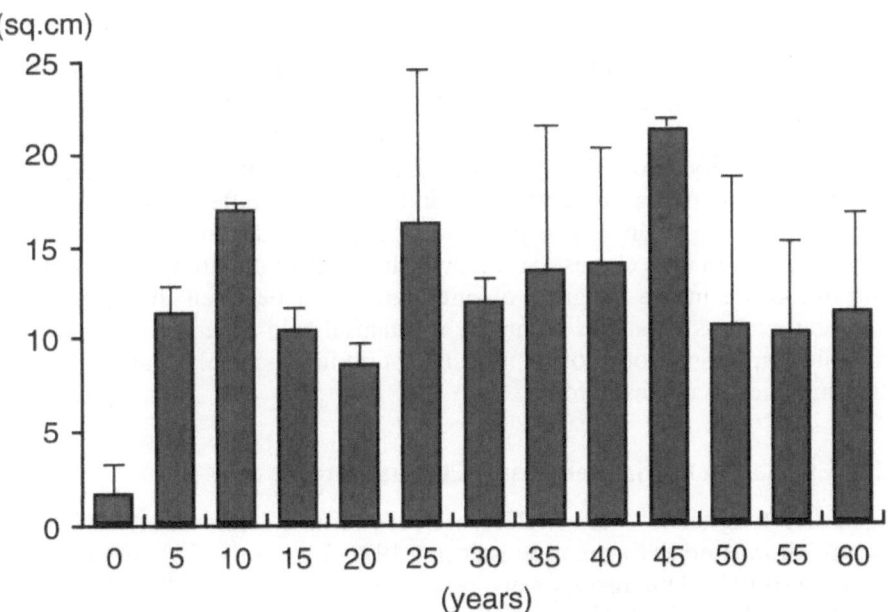

Fig. 7–2. Area of pneumatized air cells for 5-year age intervals in normal temporal bone

(sq.cm)

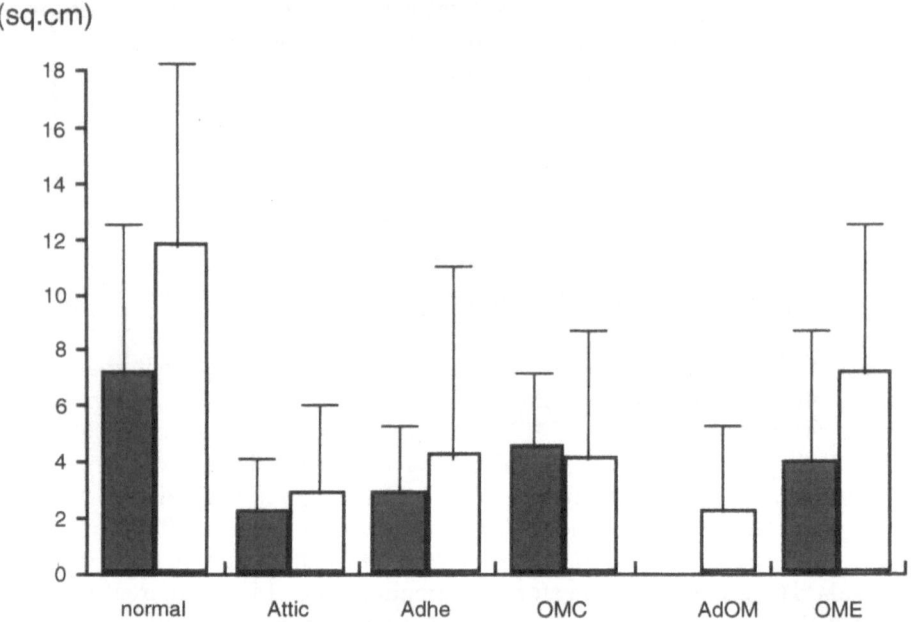

FIG. 7–3. Development of pneumatized air cells in diseases of the middle ear from childhood (*dark bars*) to adulthood (*light bars*). *Attic*, attic cholesteatoma; *Adhe*, adhesive cholesteatoma; *OMC*, otitis media chronica; *AdOM*, adhesive otitis media; *OME*, otitis media with effusion

Pneumatized areas in children under 15 and in adults with several diseases of the middle ear are shown in Fig. 7–3. The aerated area clearly increases in the normal ear and in otitis media with effusion. On the other hand, in chronic otitis media the area does not increase at all, although it is larger than those in both types of cholesteatoma. In both attic and adhesive cholesteatoma, the areas increase a little over time. The pneumatized ear in adhesive cholesteatoma is larger than that in attic cholesteatoma, which seems to indiate that there may be some difference in the progress of pneumatization between the two types of cholesteatomatous ears. For example, a mucosal fold type of partition in the tympanic diaphragm does not seem to be found in attic cholesteatoma, but it is found in adhesive cholesteatoma.

7.2.1 Exudative Otitis Media and Cholesteatoma

We studied long-term results in 245 ears with otitis media exudativa (OME) in patients who visited us for treatment during 1977–1981 and in 311 ears with OME during 1984–1988. Our results were reported in 1983 and in 1991 (Hara et al. 1983, 1991) (Table 7–1). No case of cholesteatoma was found in either study, although retracted eardrums were found in 17.1% and 14.1% of these cases,

TABLE 7-1. Long-term clinical results of otitis media exudativa (OME) reported in 1983 and 1991

Result	1977–1981	1984–1988
Nomal eardrum	116 (47.3%)	147 (47.3%)
Retraction, adhesion	42 (17.1%)	44 (14.1%)
Perforation	3 (1.2%)	7 (2.3%)
Chronic otitis media	1 (0.4%)	0
Chronic adhesive otitis	0	0
Cholesteatoma	0	0
Tubing continued		60 (19.3%)
Missed	83 (33.9%)	53 (17.0%)
Totals	245	311

TABLE 7-2. Otomicroscopic findings after OME, 1977–1986 to 1989

Finding	Pars tensa			Pars flaccida		
	No. of ears	%		No. of ears		%
Normal	156	57.8			234	86.7
Pathological	114	42.7			36	13.3
Retraction	45	28.8			36	
Calcification	39	25.0	Grade I	31		86.3
Scarring	46	29.4	II	4		11.1
Retraction	45	28.8	III	1		2.7
Adhesion	10	6.4	IV	0		0
Tubing	10	6.4				
Perforation	5	3.2				
Otorrhea	2	1.3				
Cholesteatoma	0	0				

respectively. Incidences of chronic otitis media or permanent perforation of the eardrum were negligible in both studies.

In the summer of 1989, we asked for reexamination of 535 cases diagnosed with OME during 1977–1986 in our clinic. Among them, 270 ears from 147 cases were reexamined under a surgical microscope (Table 7–2). Pathological findings were positive at the pars tensa in 42.2%, although adhesion of the pars tensa without accumulation of debris was found in 6.4%. In 36 ears (13.3%), attic retraction was found. Cases were classified according to Tos's criteria. Almost all (86%) showed grade 1 retraction. No cholesteatoma was found at either the pars flaccida or the pars tensa. Other findings were compared to those from the first visit (Table 7–3). Pneumatization was worse in cases with unfavorable outcome than in cases with favorable outcomes, and cases had been left untreated because of conditions being less severe at the first examination.

Table 7–4 lists incidences of cholesteatoma after OME. They range from 5.6%, reported by Gundersen et al. (1976), to "none," reported by Brik and Mravec

TABLE 7-3. Otological findings in OME, 1977–1986 and 1989

Finding	Unfavorable	Favorable	No treatment
A–B gap (dB)	28.6 ± 9.8	23.5 ± 9.3	16.2 ± 9.3
Tympanometry			
A	0	0.9	4.9
B	71.5	73.1	21.9
C1	28.8	16.7	58.5
C2	11.5	12.0	14.6
Pneumatization (cm²)	4.2 + 2.0	5.23 + 2.15	5.73 + 2.13
A–B gap (dB)	11.4 ± 6.5	5.2 ± 4.5	5.3 ± 4.7
Tympanometry			
A	12.0	88.3	72.4
B	28.0	0.1	1.7
C1	44.0	9.6	15.3
C2	16.0	3.0	6.9
Pneumatization (cm²)	5.33 + 3.86	10.10 + 5.90	10.2 + 6.90

TABLE 7-4. Incidence of cholesteatoma after OME as reported in the literature

Author	Year	No. of cases	No. of choles teatomas	%
Mackinnon	1971	165	8	4.8%
Mawson	1972			0.5
Kokko	1974	290	4	4.8
Tos	1976	184	2	1.1
Sadé	1976	61	2	3.2
Guderson	1976	196	11	5.6
Brik	1976	2237	0	0
Muenker	1980	1060	10	0.9
McLelland	1980	697	1	0.1
Barfoed	1980	173	0	0
Draf	1980	385	6	1.6
Karma	1982	200	2	1.0
Suzuki	1983	147	3	2.0
Onishi	1983	460	1	0.2
Yokoyama	1984	95	0	0

(1976). We therefore concluded that: (1) negative pressure in the epitympanum in OME is not so severe as to make retraction pockets deep enough for cholesteatoma to develop; and (2) OME is not the prodromal disease for attic or adhesive cholesteatoma. This conclusion may be supported also by our findings that pneumatization in OME progresses over time and is better in OME than in either type of cholesteatoma, as we reported in the preceding section.

7.2.2 Chronic Otitis Media and Cholesteatoma

The supratubal recess and its surroundings in chronic otitis media (COM) were observed in 18 ears operated on using anterior spinotomy or the usual atticotomy during tympanoplasty. The supratubal recess was found to be sound from the protympanum to through the tensor tympani mucosal fold, using angled sounds graduated in 1-mm increments at the tip. The anterior attic bony plate was also measured using graduated sounds in front of the head of the malleus. Mucosal folds were determined to be of "unknown" condition when it was not clear whether they were perforated by exploration with a probe or by some surgical procedures. Our results, reported in 1991, are shown in Table 7–5a and 7–5b.

Patients' ages ranged from 9 to 63 years, with an average of 35.5 years. The pneumatized area measured on Schuller's x-ray films ranged from 2.1 cm to 16.0 cm, with an average of 7.4 cm. Among them, attic retraction was recognized in three ears; two ears had grade II and one a grade I retraction, by Tos's classification. The size of the supratubal recess was large in six, medium in four,

TABLE 7–5a. Surgical findings in the supratubal recess and its surroundings in chronic otitis media

No.	1	2	3	4	5	6	7	8	9	10	11	12	13	14	15	16	17	18
Age	63	47	13	55	60	60	9	21	40	61	44	54	53	12	12	11	13	11
Sex	F	F	F	F	F	M	F	F	M	F	F	F	F	M	M	M	F	M
Attic R			T?								T2	T1						
Pneumat.	5	13	2	16	2	2	13	1	20	13	4	2	2			18	7	5
STR	s	l	m	l	s	s	m	m	l	s	m	s	s	l	l	l	l	m
AABP																		
(l)	l	m	m	s	m	l	l	m	m	s	l	l	s	s	s		l	
(w)	m	m	m	tn	m	tk	tn	tk	tn	tn	tk	tk	tn				tk	
AAMF	+	−	+	−	−			−	−	+	+	−	−	−	−	−	−	−
S.M.	+	−	−	+	−		−	−	−	−	−	+	−	+	+	−	−	−
Glue	+	−	−	−	−	−	−	−	−	−	+	+	−	−	−	−	−	−
Ty. Isth	−			−	−	−	−	−			−	−						−

Attic R, Attic retraction; Pneumat., pneumatization; STR, supratubal recess; s, small; m, medium; l, large; AABP, anterior attic bony plate; (l), length; s, short; m, medium; l, long; (w), width; tn, thin; tk, thick; m, medium; AAMF, anterior attic mucosal fold; +, closure; −, perforated; S.M., swelling of attic mucosa; Ty. Isth., tympanic isthmus.

TABLE 7–5b. Surgical findings in the supratubal recess and its surroundings in 18 ears with chronic otitis media

Age	9–36 years old		Average, 35.5 years	
Sex	F, 12 ears		M, 6 ears	
Pneumatization	2.1–16.0 mm^2		Average, 7.4 mm^2	
Attic retraction	Grade II, 2 ears		Grade I, 1 ear	
Supratubal recess	Large, 6	Medial, 4	Small, 7	Unknown, 0
Anterior attic bony plate	Large, 6	Medial, 5	Small, 4	Unknown, 2
	Thick, 5	Medial, 4	Thin, 5	Unknown, 4
Tensor mucosal fold	Perforated, 16	Intact, 0	Unknown, 2	
Anterior attic mucosal fold	Perforated, 12	Intact, 4	Unknown, 2	
Tympanic isthmus	Open, 9	Closed, 0	Unknown, 9	
Mesotympanic mucosa	Pathological, 8	Normal, 10		
Attic mucosa	Pathological, 5	Normal, 12	Unknown, 1	
Glue	Retention, 3	None, 15		

and small in seven ears. The anterior attic bony plate was long (3mm) in six, medium (2mm) in five, short (1mm) in four, and unknown in two ears. It was thick in five, of medium thickness in four, thin in five, and of unknown thickness in four ears.

The tensor tympani mucosal fold was perforated in 16 ears; its condition in the other 2 ears was unknown. The anterior attic mucosal fold was perforated in 12 ears, not perforated in 4 ears, and of unknown condition in 2 ears. The tympanic isthmus was open in 9 ears and of unknown condition in 9 ears; there was no case with definite closure. The mucosa in the mesotympanum was pathologically edematous in 8 ears and almost normal in 12 ears. In the attic, the mucosa was pathological in 5 and normal in 12 ears. Retention of glue in the tympanic cavity was observed in 3 ears with edematous mucosa. Three ears with attic retractions had a medium-sized or small supratubal recess with a long, thick, anterior attic bony plate and an intact (not perforated) anterior attic mucosal fold; their pneumatized areas were 2–3 cm. All other cases, however, had perforated mucosal folds.

Histological studies of temporal bones with COM were also performed by one of our team at the Minnesota Temporal Bone Laboratory (Morimitsu, 1991). It was observed in many cases of COM that exudate from the attic flowed into the

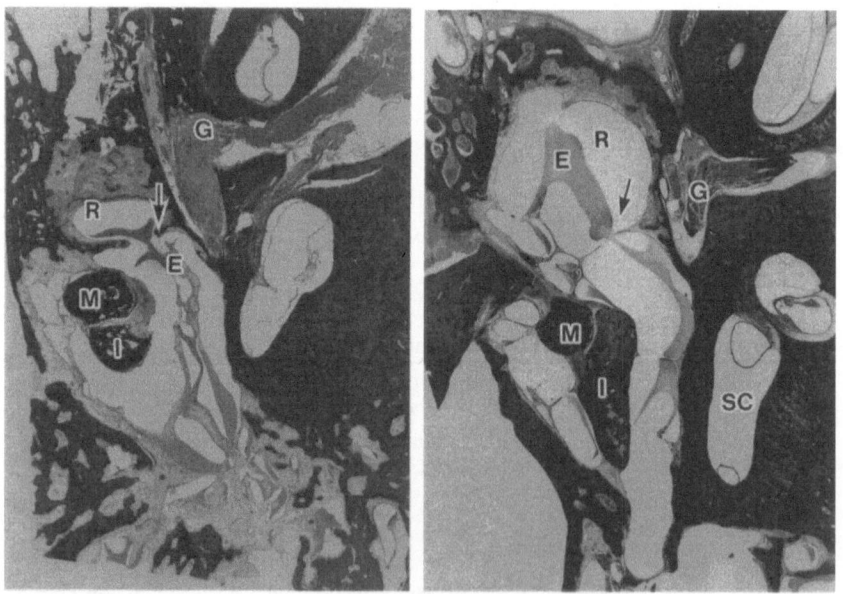

a   b

Fig. 7–4a,b. Histopathology of otitis media chronica. a Exudate flows into the supratubal recess through the perforated anterior attic bony plate (*arrow*). b Exudate flows into the supratubal recess through the perforated anterior attic mucosal fold (*arrow*). R, supratubal recess; E, exudate; M, malleus; I, incus; G, geniculate ganglion; SC, semicircular canal

supratubal recess through a defect in the anterior attic bony plate (Fig. 7–4a) or a perforation of the anterior attic mucosal fold (Fig. 7–4b). These findings indicate that exudate flows out from the epitympanum into the mesotympanum through the tympanic isthmus or into the protympanum through perforated superior and inferior partitions in the supratubal recess.

During the past three decades, we have treated more than 2000 cases of COM in our clinic, but only 1 such case (Morimitsu and Kano, 1990) developed attic cholesteatoma after long-lasting COM. This patient was a 37-year-old man who at first had a small perforation in the pars tensa with a grade I attic retraction. Two years later he visited us again because of acute exacerbation with otorrhea from a perforation in the pars tensa. At that time the attic retraction had a small cholesteatoma that could be removed using a suction tube. The perforation in his eardrum was closed during conservative treatment. Three years later he came back with increased loss of hearing. He was operated on because of a large attic cholesteatoma in which a plate-type partition was found. In our experience, therefore, it is very rare for cholesteatoma to develop in cases of COM, although the development of pneumatization in both diseases is almost equal.

From the findings we observed in COM we concluded that: (1) the anatomical condition of the tympanic diaphragm in COM is different from that in attic

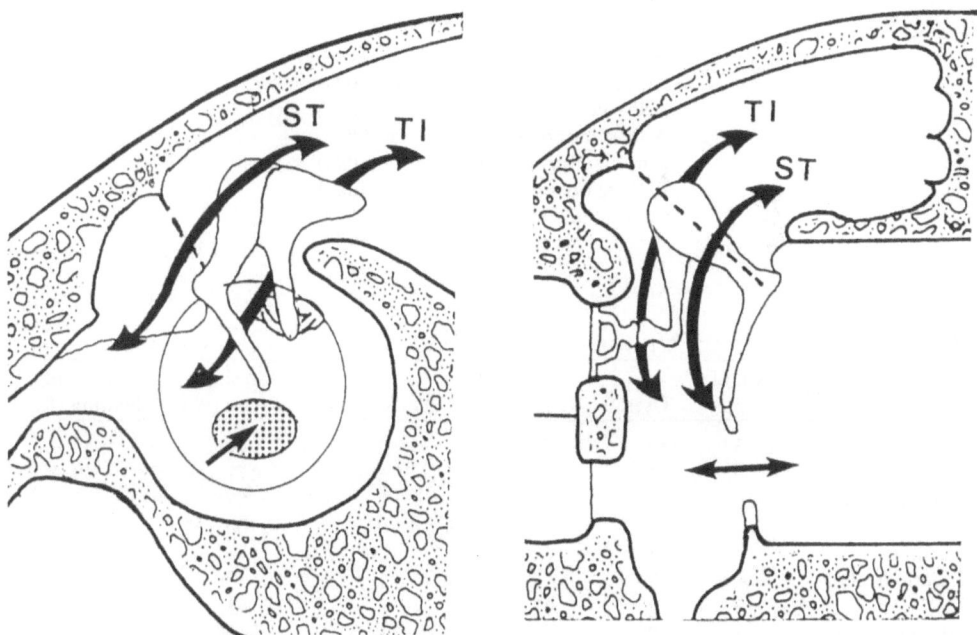

Fig. 7–5a,b. Ventilation through the tympanic diaphragm in otitis media chronica (left middle ear). **a** Side view. **b** Frontal view. *ST*, ventilation through the supratubal recess; *TI*, ventilation through the tympanic isthmus; *arrow*, tympanic perforation

cholesteatoma, i.e., it is a membranous tympanic diaphragm with a patent tympanic isthmus and a perforated anterior attic mucosal fold; and (2) cases of COM with attic retraction may develop cholesteatoma when acutely exacerbated after tympanoplasty or on closure of a perforation of the eardrum, because in such cases the supratubal ventilating route is closed and function in the eustachian tube is impaired. Our surgical anatomical findings in COM are illustrated in Fig. 7–5.

7.2.3 Adhesive Otitis Media and Cholesteatoma

Almost all cases of adhesive otitis media continue as they are without developing adhesive cholesteatoma. To make clear the reasons, Makino et al. (1955) studied 88 ears with adhesive otitis media operated on in our clinic during 1978 to 1994. They consisted of 64 ears from male patients and 24 ears from female patients. Ages ranged from 5 to 67 years. Otoscopic findings in the opposite ears are shown in Table 7–6. About 50% of the cases had several pathological findings, indicating that patients with adhesive otitis media have some systemic causative factors (e.g., anemia, leukopenia, hypo-gammaglobulinemia, poor immunological resistance, sinusitis, tonsillitis, or adenoids) for diseases of the middle ear.

TABLE 7–6. Otoscopic findings in opposite ears

Otoscopic findings	Ears
Normal	44 (50%)
Adhesive otitis media	14 (16%)
Adhesive cholesteatoma	8 (9%)
Chronic otitis media	9 (10%)
Radical operations	9 (10%)
Otitis media eudativa	4 (5%)

TABLE 7–7. Procedures against readhesion and their results

Procedures	No. of ears	Uses	Readhesion	Perforation	Success, cavity (%)	Rates of hearing (%)
None	23	10	11	2	44	65
Gelfilm	35	14	6	4	71	49
Silicon block	14	8	6	0	57	43
Antrum mucosa	5	5	0	0	100	60
Cartilage	4	3	1	0	75	75
Lateral healing	4	2	1	1	50	50
Gelfoam	3	2	1	0	67	67
Nasal mucosa	2	0	1	1	0	50
Total removal	2	1	0	1	50	50
Totals	92[a]	61%	29%	10%	61%	55

[a] Two procedures were used in two ears, so the total number is larger.

TABLE 7-8. Surgical findings in the mastoid and success rates in myringoplasty

Findings	No. of ears	Success rate	Readhesion	Perforation
Normal	7	4 (57%)	3	0
Thick mucosa	17	13 (77%)	4	0
Full granulation	9	3 (33%)	4	2
Cholesterin granuloma	12	5 (42%)	4	3
Exudate	6	4 (67%)	2	0
Small antrum	3	2 (67%)	0	1

All cases underwent tympanoplasty, also combined with intact canal wall mastoidectomy in 54 cases. Nine procedures were used against readhesion of the new eardrum (Table 7-7). Readhesion of the new eardrum was observed in 29%, but neither adhesive cholesteatoma nor retraction pockets into the epitympanum by the new eardrum were found postoperatively. In 86%, the tympanic orifice of the eustachian tube was patent, and the rate of success in myringoplasty was 60%. There were no differences in success rates between those with open or with closed orifices of the eustachian tube. The tympanic isthmus was open in 24% and closed in 76%, and the success rates for myringoplasty were 80% and 53%, respectively.

Surgical findings in mastoidectomy are shown in Table 7-8. In all cases except the group with full granulation, one of the ventilating routes (through the supratubal recess or through the tympanic isthmus) was patent. Granulation tissue or cholesterin granuloma in the mastoid was removed, but the mucosa was retained as much as possible. The best results were obtained in the group with thick mucosa, and the poorest in the group with full granuloma.

From our findings we concluded (1) that adhesive cholesteatoma had not developed postoperatively even when a new eardrum had readhered on the promontory because of a patent tympanic isthmus or a supratubal ventilating route (membranous tympanic diaphragm); and (2) that anterior tympanotomy, therefore, should change adhesive cholesteatoma to adhesive otitis media in which recurrence of cholesteatoma is impossible even though postoperative aeration of the new tympanic cavity cannot be maintained. Our surgical anatomical findings are illustrated in Fig. 7-6.

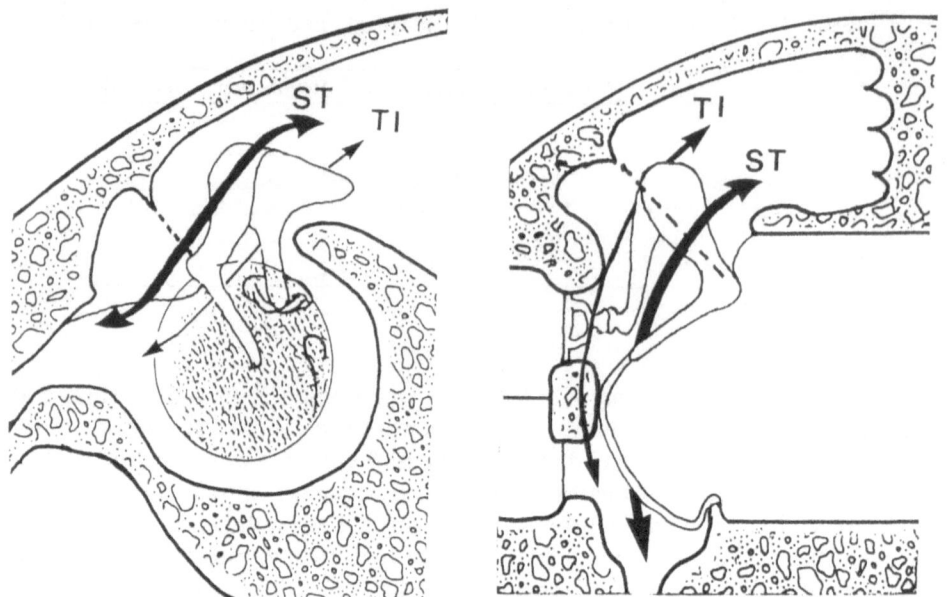

Fig. 7–6a,b. Ventilation through the tympanic diaphragm in adhesive otitis media (left middle ear). **a** Side view. **b** Frontal view. *ST*, ventilation through the supratubal recess; *TI*, ventilation through the tympanic isthmus

7.3 Developmental Processes of Attic Cholesteatoma

The developmental process of acquired attic cholesteatoma can be explained as follows: (Fig. 7–7).

1. Pneumatization of the temporal bone in babyhood is inhibited by unknown etiological factors, probably acute otitis media or an unknown congenital disposition, and thus the tympanic diaphragm remains as a bony tympanic diaphragm without a ventilating route through the supratubal recess.

2. In acute otitis media, the tympanic isthmuses are closed by swollen mucous membrane and thick mucoid exudate; thus, negative pressure develops in the epitympanum for long periods even though the eustachian tube may recover patency and the mesotympanum may recover to normal pressure.

3. The flaccid membrane then retracts into Prussak's space and further into the epitympanum, forming a deep retraction pocket. According to our study, in one-third of cases Prussak's space has only a single communicating route to the epitympanum. In such cases, negative pressure can develop in Prussak's space alone even though the tympanic isthmus may be open, and thus a retraction pocket may localize in Prussak's space alone.

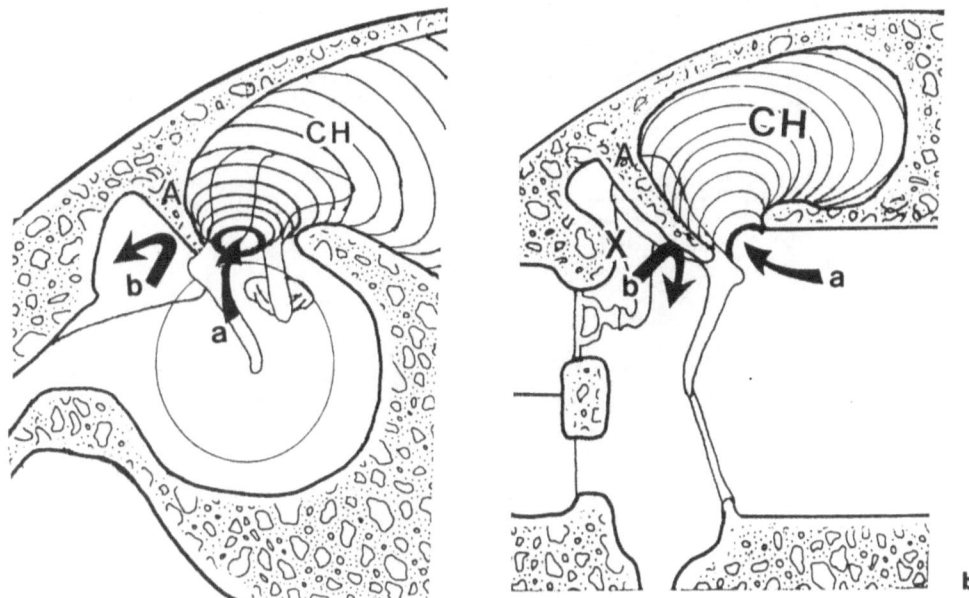

Fig. 7–7a,b. Development of an attic cholesteatoma. **a** Side view. **b** Frontal view. *CH*, cholesteatoma; *A*, osseous or bony tympanic diaphragm; *X*, closure of the tympanic isthmus; *Arrow a*, attic retraction followed by cholesteatoma; *arrow b*, blockage of ventilation through the supratubal recess

4. At the introitus of the pocket, migration of epidermis in and out gives rise to a "traffic jam," and desquamated debris accumulates in the pocket, forming a small cholesteatomatous mass.

5. Bacterial infection in the accumulated desquamation promotes further proliferation of keratinized epidermis in the pocket, and thus the cholesteatoma gradually expands over the ossicles into the epitympanum.

6. The enlarged cholesteatoma acts as an obstructor of the ventilating routes in the tympanic diaphragm, causing long-lasting, severe negative pressure in the atticomastoid cavity. In this condition, cholesteatoma grows rapidly into the whole atticomastoid space.

7.4 Developmental Processes of Adhesive Cholesteatoma

The developmental processes in acquired adhesive cholesteatoma can be explained as illustrated in Fig. 7–8.

1. The bony tympanic diaphragm in acute otitis media is the same as that in attic cholesteatoma.

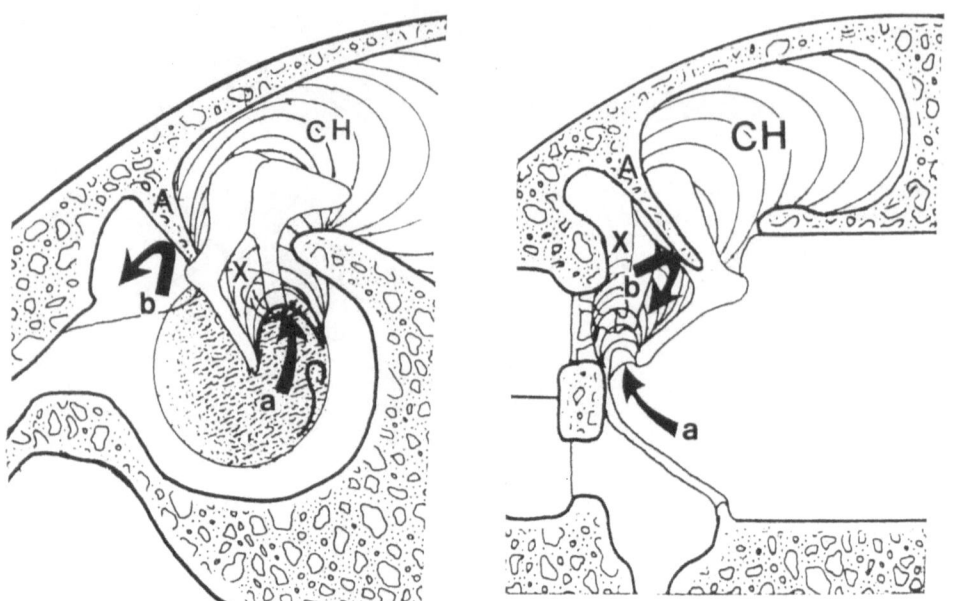

a   **b**

Fig. 7–8a,b. Development of an adhesive cholesteatoma. **a** Side view. **b** Frontal view. *CH*, cholesteatoma; *A*, osseous or bony tympanic diaphragm; *X*, closure of the tympanic isthmus; *arrow a*, retraction of posterior superior quadrant; *arrow b*, blockage of ventilation through the supratubal recess

2. After acute otitis media with long-lasting tubal stenosis, the eardrum adheres on the promontory. Especially, the posterior superior quadrant of the adhered eardrum blocks all or part of the oval window, the tympanic sinus, and the introitus of the posterior tympanic isthmus at the level of the incudostapedial joint.

3. By acute exacerbation or secondary acute otitis media, the swollen mucosa and thick mucoid exudate assist in blocking the anterior tympanic isthmus, the only ventilation route between the eustachian tube and the atticomastoid cavity.

4. Negative pressure develops in the atticomastoid cavity and causes a deep retraction pocket from the adhered posterior superior quadrant of the eardrum, which is thin and atrophic.

5. Cholesteatoma thus develops and breaks the incudostapedial joint, then grows into the atticomastoid cavity through the patent posterior tympanic isthmus under the ossicles.

6. If the tympanic diaphragm is membranous and the posterior tympanic isthmus is closed, the cholesteatoma remains only in the oval window niche or the tympanic sinus for long periods, because negative pressure does not develop in the atticomastoid cavity. The absence of negative pressure means that there is no driving force for growth of cholesteatoma into the atticomastoid cavity.

7. In rare cases, adhesive cholesteatoma develops into the supratubal recess or the premalleolar space from the anterior superior quadrant of the adhered eardrum. In such cases, a ventilating route is patent from the eustachian tube to the atticomastoid cavity through the posterior tympanic isthmus.

Finally, we concluded that the real pathogenesis of acquired cholesteatoma lies in the bony tympanic diaphragm, which is a sequela of poor pneumatization of the temporal bone. If the bony tympanic diaphragm has not been demolished in cholesteatomatous ears operated on using the canal-up method, recurrence of cholesteatoma is inevitable. For complete cure of acquired cholesteatoma, it is necessary not only to eradicate the pathological tissue but also to change the bony tympanic diaphragm to a membranous diaphragm using anterior tympanotomy.

References

Barfoed C, Rosberg J (1980) Secretory otitis media: long-term observation after treatment with grommets. Arch Otolaryngol 106:553–556

Bezold F (1908) Textbook of otology (trans. by Holinger H) Colgrove, Chicago, p 189

Brik HG, Mravec JT (1976) Myringotomy for middle ear effusions: results of two-year study. Ann Otol Rhinol Laryngol 85(suppl 25):263–267

Draf W (1980) Insertion of ventilation tubes into the middle ear: results, complications— a seven-year review. Ann Rhinol Laryngol 89(suppl 68):303–307

Gunderson T, Tonning F-M (1976) Ventilation tubes in the middle ear: long-term observations. Arch Otolaryngol 102:198–199

Habermann J (1889) Zur Entstehung des Cholesteatoms des Mittelohrs. Arch Ohrenheilk 27:42–46

Hara Y, Kano K, Masuda M, Toyama K, Matsuda K, Tsuboi Y, Morimitsu T (1991) Clinical results of ventilation tube therapy of otitis media with effusion (in Japanese with English abstract). Otol Fukuoka 37:557–561

Hara Y, Hidaka S, Tono T, Makino K, Kasano F, Ide M, Enatsu K, Ushisako Y, Morimitsu T (1983) Clinical results of secretory otitis media (in Japanese). Clin Otol Jpn 10:266–267

Karma P (1982) Long-term results of tympanotomy treatment in chronic secretory otitis media. Acta Otolaryngol (Stockh) Suppl 386:163–165

Kokko E (1976) Clinical results and complications of tympanostomy. Ann Otol Rhinol Laryngol 85(suppl 25):277–279

Mackinnon DM (1971) The sequel to myringotomy for exudative otitis media. J Laryngol Otol 82:773–793

Makino K, Inaba J, Tono T, Morimitsu T (1995) Evaluation of surgical procedure for adhesive cholesteatoma (in Japanese with English abstract). Otol Jpn 5:26–31

Mawson SR, Fagan P (1972) Tympanic effusion in children: long-term results of treatment by myringotomy, aspiration, and indwelling tubes (grommets). J Laryngol Otol 86:105–119

McLelland CA (1980) Incidence of complications from use of tympanotomy tubes. Arch Otolaryngol 106:97–99

Miyanaga S, Morimitsu T (1989) A planimetric study of temporal bone pneumatization in cholesteatoma. In: Tos M, Thomsen J, Peitersen E (eds) Cholesteatoma and mastoid surgery. Kugler Ghedini, Amsterdam, pp 259–263

Morimitsu T (1991) Etiology of middle ear cholesteatoma (in Japanese with English abstract) Otol Fukuoka 37:271–405

Morimitsu T, Kano K (1990) Prevention of cholesteatoma: is it possible or not? (in Japanese). Otolaryngol Head Neck Surg 16:28–32

Muenker G (1980) Results after treatment of otitis media with effusion. Ann Otol Rhinol Laryngol 89(suppl 68):308–311

Onishi T (1983) Development of cholesteatoma from otitis media with effusion (in Japanese with English abstract). Otolaryngol Tokyo 55:691–696

Proctor B (1989) Surgical anatomy of the ear. Blackwell, Oxford

Sadé J (1976) Atelectasis and secretory otitis media. Ann Otol Rhinol Laryngol 85:66–73

Suzuki M, Modera K, Yamada O (1983) Long-term observation of secretory otitis media in children (in Japanese). Clin Otol 10:240–241

Tos M, Poulsen G (1976) Secretory otitis media: late results of treatment with grommets. Arch Otolaryngol 102:672–675

Wendt H (1873) Desquamative Entzundung des Mittelohrs. Arch Ohrenheilk 14:428–432

Wittmaack K (1933) Wie entstehet ein genuines Cholesteatoma? Arch Ohren-Nasen-Kehlkophheilkunde 137:306–332

Yokoyama T (1984) Treatment in secretory otitis media—how to choose grommets (in Japanese). Otolaryngol Tokyo 56:833–841

Index